The FAD-PROOF Diet

Greg Green, DC

About the Author

Greg Green is a writer and chiropractor living in Houston, Texas. His first career was teaching writing and English literature. Besides his private practice, Greg runs the site N1Experiment.com, where he writes about his experiments about everything from his weight-loss strategies to improving his singing.

Greg enjoys playing music, cooking, eating what he cooks, and spending time with his family.

Table of Contents

ONE
Fad-Diet Checklist

Most of the big fads and trends in the dieting world are oppressively strict. And the evidence shows that people who follow an "all or nothing" approach to dieting have the highest rate of re-gain. The process commonly called "flexible dieting" is the opposite of the fad diets that are popular now. The whole point of flexible dieting, as the name might imply, is that you have true flexibility when it comes to everything from what you eat to when you eat it. More on that in the next chapters.

Let's examine some common themes of dieting fads. Think of these points as ways to know your enemy. The overarching theme of all fad diets is that they somehow trick their adherents into eating less. And when people have success, especially initially, they want to tell everyone they know about how awesome their diet is. Knowing someone who has had success with weight loss can be especially compelling when considering a program for yourself. The following points can help you decide if you should take the plunge.

First up—is there true scientific validation of the program or protocol? Many diets have a "guru" or person claiming superior knowledge attached to them, and many of these gurus sound "science-y" when they're explaining their ideas. But what is the consensus of the scientific community at large?

Admittedly, figuring out the consensus of the scientific community can be a challenge. Often, the guru in question may even have a string of letters after their name to lend credibility to their claims. However, sometimes the best way to figure out their motivation is to follow the money. Are they selling you something? Especially something you must keep continually buying? Buyer beware.

Guru-led diet fads almost universally use testimonials to support the idea that their diet is the one that works. Testimonials are powerful when it comes to human behavior. We tend to do what our friends say far more often than doing what research tells us.

One of the big secret weapons in the guru diet toolbox is using a technique called "appeals to authority." You've seen it plenty of times—a celebrity or doctor or, even worse, a doctor-celebrity, who says that *this* diet is the latest and greatest and newest and best.

Never mind that the average celebrity knows nothing about biochemistry or the psychology behind dieting. Hey, they looked great on the red-carpet last week—good enough, right? No. It's their job to look awesome, and they often make a lot of money doing it. Also, there's just no way to know what their actual regimen looks like. The diet they're espousing may be much different from their personal reality.

If a celebrity is telling you to put butter in your coffee or do some kind of cleansing enema, just keep on trucking.

Next—are you being told you must eat a certain food to have weight loss success? What about the opposite, being instructed to stay away from major food groups? Any time there is a rigid stance on what you can eat or not eat you may be following a fad diet. Especially if you're being advised to stay away from an entire group of macronutrients—that is to say, carbs, protein, or fat. (More on that later.)

I'll be the first to tell you that to lose fat you'll have to restrict calories. Restricting calories, by its very definition, means you'll have to restrict some macronutrient intake. But there's a big difference between simple "restriction" and "extreme restriction." Again, staying flexible is the key to long-term diet success.

If you are being told that you can lose all the weight you want by following a few "simple" but rigid rules, you are being set up to do something unsustainable. Anyone can follow extremely rigid rules for a finite amount of time. But when you arrive at your goal and haven't learned how to stay at that level without following the guidelines that made getting there in the first place pure hell, well, you're going to have nowhere to go but back to the same starting weight or worse.

Many of these diet fads create scenarios where adherents deprive themselves of vital nutrients in the quest to improve their health. Be suspicious of any guru telling you that you "only have to" eat this, avoid that, or buy this supplement. Especially if they have a celebrity or two backing them up and a website loaded with testimonials.

With the flexible dieting approach, as you're about to find out, there's no need to categorize foods as good or bad ever again. There will be room for the occasional minor indulgence. You can lose the weight you desire in a systematic way based on real science and real results.

All you have to do is keep reading.

TWO
Common Misconceptions of Dieters

I think I'm in starvation mode because I'm barely eating anything and I'm still not losing weight.

There's a trend in popular dieting culture to think that if the body is deprived of calories long enough that weight loss will stop, or even reverse, because of something commonly called "starvation mode."

Here's the good news: starvation mode doesn't exist. In every metabolic ward study, meaning a study conducted in a clinic ward where caloric intake is strictly controlled, people lose weight—every time, without fail. The fact is, you can't stop physics. The energy balance equation, the relationship between your body's energy intake and its output trumps all, including hormones, starvation mode, or anything else. This is good news because it puts the power back in your hands.

You have ultimate control over your caloric intake. Now, I'm not saying this is easy. It can be incredibly challenging to take control of the fork. We live in a society where tasty, calorie-dense food surrounds us. There are shows on television where people compete to make the best cupcakes. We are surrounded by the truthful message that eating is a pleasure and a right. And we all know it's a necessity.

If you're an alcoholic, you can stop drinking (anytime I want!) and avoid all alcohol. But you cannot avoid all food, since you must eat to stay alive. Add social situations, work lunches, and boredom to the mix, and it can make for a challenging situation to get your food intake under control. But you're not in starvation mode.

The fact is, people are very good at forgetting the nibble or two they ate here and there. A study from the US National Library of Medicine entitled "Discrepancy between self-reported and actual caloric intake and exercise in obese subjects" showed that people are inherently bad at tracking their own calories.

The conclusion of the study states, "The failure of some obese subjects to lose weight while eating a diet they report as low in calories is due to an energy intake substantially higher than reported and an overestimation of physical activity, not to an abnormality in thermogenesis." In other words, people overestimated how many calories they were burning and underestimated how much they were eating in the first place.

The first step to getting a handle on this "tracking issue" is knowing that many people naturally suck when it comes to tracking, and then resolving to do better than most people. It can be done. I promise.

This is not to say that being in a calorie deficit for an extended period of time will not make the body respond hormonally—it will. Your body doesn't like extended dieting. It will try to make you eat more. But you can't deny physics.

I'm exercising every day and I still can't lose the weight.

Another common misconception is that increased activity, especially purposeful goal-oriented exercise like group classes and lifting weights, is an effective way to burn off excess calories. It's not. Weight loss is much easier to handle through diet than through exercise.

It is far easier to track how many calories are in a food that you want to eat than it is to calculate how much you are really burning during an activity. And like the study I mentioned above said, people are way more likely to overestimate their activity than keep an accurate record.

But it's not just the overestimation that hurts them. Another thing that happens when people exercise a lot is that they get hungrier. They think, "Hey, I worked out, I can eat a little more." You see where this is going.

In addition, for some people exercise slows something called Non-Exercise Activity Thermogenesis: NEAT. NEAT is all the daily moving around and fidgeting that people naturally do. People who seem to have higher metabolisms often have a very high rate of NEAT working for them. They just can't sit still for very long. They burn calories at a higher rate because they are always moving, but intense exercise can blunt that effect. Bottom line: fat loss starts with your diet.

⟶ That's not to say that you can't use a little cardio to shave off a few hundred calories here and there. Sometimes you're just not going to be willing to eat less than you already are. But get your head around the diet part of the equation first.

"Clean" versus "dirty" foods

Speaking of diet, one common misconception among dieters is the concept of "clean" versus "dirty" foods.

Here's what you need to know—as long as you're not overeating in terms of total calories, it really doesn't matter which foods you eat when it comes to losing body fat. Many (many!) of the health benefits people see from following whichever fat-loss diet they choose come from the fat loss itself, not the actual diet they used to lose that fat.

Some people have great success using a diet that gives a general framework of rules leading to eating fewer calories overall. The Paleo Diet is an example. People across the country lose fat on the Paleo Diet and find their blood lipid markers improved in the process. They jump to the conclusion that the diet itself has led to improved health, not realizing that the results came from dieting in general. For example, nutrition professor Mark Haub, a researcher at Kansas State University, lost 27 pounds over ten weeks in 2010 eating almost exclusively crap that he bought at a gas station including

Twinkies and chips. He diligently tracked his intake. At the end of his gas-station diet experiment his blood labs had all improved.

Am I telling you food quality doesn't matter at all? No, I'm not. I am telling you that you can make some significant strides in improving your health by simply eating less of the foods you already prefer. There are some other strategies, too, which is why this book has more than one chapter. But the idea that there are "bad" or "dirty" foods needs to be erased from your mindset right now.

Another example of a food that gets put in the "bad camp" (as opposed to band camp) is sugar. Sugar has no micronutrients and is easy to overeat, but that doesn't mean it can't find an occasional place in your diet. Research bears this out, as mentioned in the study entitled "Metabolic and behavioral effects of a high-sucrose diet during weight loss."

In this study all the meals were provided for the participants by the researchers. One group was fed a very high sugar diet and one group ate almost no sugar at all. Carbohydrate content and overall calories were identical for both groups.

At the end of the study no significant difference was shown between the group that ate sugar and the group that limited it. Here's a quote from the study itself: "Results showed that a high sucrose content in a hypoenergetic, low-fat diet did not adversely affect weight loss, metabolism, plasma lipids, or emotional affect." In plain English, that means that as long as you're eating fewer calories, you're going to lose weight without negative consequences to your health even if you have some sugar in your diet.

> One thing that happens when you start tracking what you eat is that you'll find that you can fit things like sugar in here and there, but you won't feel as satisfied. Tracking will help you choose more filling, nutritious foods so you don't feel as hungry all the time. But still, sometimes you gotta eat some ice cream.

You can always start micromanaging your food choices later when you want to fine-tune and optimize your health. But, start where you are. The big reason fad diets are bad for people is that they are unsustainable for most, and once the diet ends and regular eating habits are resumed the train goes off the tracks quickly, which leads to the dreaded "yo-yo dieting" effect.

And that leads us to our final common misconception: damaged metabolism.

Broken metabolism

I've had more than my share of people tell me that they must have a slow metabolism because they're "barely eating anything and still not losing weight." A small car burns less fuel than a big truck, and it's the same with people. A larger person, whether their weight is stored in excess body fat or excess muscle, has a faster metabolism than a smaller person. But someone who has dieted off fifty pounds only to regain the weight and then some may find that their resting metabolic rate is slightly lower, in fact, than someone of the same weight who has never attempted to diet.

This doesn't mean you can't lose weight. It might mean losing weight will be a little harder, but it can be done using the guidelines in this book. A quick hint: The more nutrient-dense but calorie-poor foods you eat, the more you will be able to control your appetite. Managing your appetite is the way to win the battle over and over again that will eventually lead you to win the weight-loss war.

Other people believe they've been eating so few calories that their body is attempting to hold on to its fat stores, and therefore they can't lose weight (as in the "starvation mode" above). Sometimes they have the feeling they're putting on even more fat because their body is storing any foods they do eat as additional adipose tissue, and it's their busted metabolism creating the problem. But here's what is happening every time, without fail: the person in question is eating more than they think. People eating more than they think is a theme running throughout this book. Why? Because eating more than we think we are eating is the number one reason we can't lose weight.

THREE
The Fundamentals of Flexible Dieting

People follow fad diets, which are usually too restrictive and unsustainable, because they don't know the fundamentals of flexible dieting. And when you don't know the basics, it's easy to buy into the false logic of the New Best Diet Ever found in the magazines or that your friends are talking about on social media. So, we're going to dive right into the basics now and fill in the finer details as we get into this book. The biggest "advanced tactic" you can learn is that there are no advanced tactics to worry about, unless you're trying to get stage-ready for a bodybuilding show.

Below is a short list of the fundamentals:

1. Caloric intake dictates fat gain or fat loss. Allow me to make a bold statement: people's success with fad diets is due to the fact that these diets force behavior changes that lower their overall daily caloric intake. Period.

2. There are advantages to prioritizing specific macronutrients (that is, protein, carbs, and fat) when trying to eat fewer overall calories. Protein, especially, is nearly magical when used in creating a calorie deficit without the dieter feeling too deprived.

3. Exercise is a horrible way to create a calorie deficit, but it's a great way to send the signal to the body for muscle retention. You want to retain the muscle mass you already have when you're dieting, so you'll lose the fat and keep the muscle. Without muscle retention, you'll become "skinny fat," which you probably don't want.

4. Focus on the daily habits that will help you make progress, instead of focusing on the end goal. You have to learn to embrace the journey, not the destination.

Instead of fad diets that very seldom lead to long-term weight loss, Flexible Dieting is the method that offers the most success. To the more evidence-based community of fitness and dieting writers, Flexible Dieting has become one of the standard ways to describe the process this book details. To start, Flexible Dieting allows the dieter flexibility with their food choices, which will in turn make it much easier to stick to the process of losing weight. Because getting there is much easier for most people than staying there, if you can stick to the dieting process during the "losing" part of your fat-loss journey, it'll be much easier to maintain that process once you've reached your desired weight.

Our bodies are wired to store fat. But after a diet, hormonal shifts can start a war with hunger which often leads to the phenomenon known as "yo-yo dieting": losing a bunch of weight, and then gaining it all back and then some. We don't want that, so we're going to approach weight loss in a smart, strategic way that will enable you to coast into your desired weight and stay there while slowly increasing your overall calories until you hit maintenance intake.

The first significant step is to adjust your expectations. Most people want their fat loss to happen yesterday. That kind of thinking is what leads people to jump onto the latest fad diet that promises rapid fat loss just in time for their next class reunion or summer at the beach. Don't fall for it. Learning and then mastering the fundamentals of flexible dieting will give you the keys to the fat-loss kingdom without resorting to extremes. ("The extremes" are anything that equals massive deprivation or following super-strict rules about what you can or can't eat as well as when you can eat.)

Yes, you will need to learn the difference between being hungry and just being bored. You will have to learn to live, and even thrive, with a bit of hunger pecking away at you sometimes. But if you do this right, you can be a leaner, healthier, more in-control version of yourself within the next year or so. A reasonable amount of fat loss to expect is anywhere from half a pound to a pound a week. Maybe a little bit more if you have a lot to lose.

> I hate to be the bearer of bad news, but sometimes, when you're trying to eat less, you will be hungry.

You'll also have to trust the process, because fat loss isn't a linear progression. The leaner you get, the more you'll have to coax your body to drop down to the next level. You will find that sometimes the scale won't budge for a few days or even a week or more. You'll feel moments of desperation when this happens. And then you'll be shocked when it seems like you suddenly dropped 5-7 pounds overnight. Understanding the fundamentals is where the magic happens. Let's look at the fundamentals like they're a pyramid, with the base of the pyramid being the most critical factor, then moving up by order of importance.

Before diving into this idea, I'd like to acknowledge Eric Helms as the inspiration and brains behind the pyramid concept. Eric is a PhD, bodybuilder, and science-based stallion in the field of body composition and training. He has a fantastic breakdown of his pyramid on YouTube. The pyramid he came up with is in my opinion the best way to understand the basics. Many fitness and weight loss writers out there have taken to using his method of explaining the basics. Eric doesn't know me from Adam, but, Eric, if you happen to read this—thanks for the inspiration, man. Anyway, back to the pyramid.

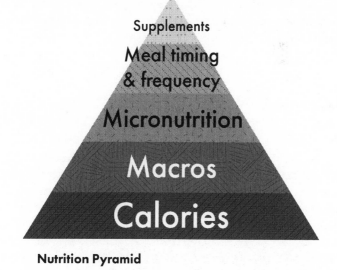

Supplements

Meal timing & frequency

Micronutrition

Macros

Calories

Nutrition Pyramid

At the base of our pyramid, the foundation, is your overall caloric intake. If you decrease total calories without changing one other thing the needle on the scale will start to move downward. Total intake is the most critical part of the puzzle. It's simple physics.

The next level up the pyramid is macronutrient intake. If you've been dieting off and on for years, have a general awareness of the calories you consume and are wanting to fine-tune your intake, tracking your macro intake is the next logical step. All the calories you eat are composed of protein, carbohydrates, or fats in some combination. Tweaking that combination can make it easier for you to stay satisfied and full while dieting, give you energy in the gym, and make this whole journey far less miserable.

Although it's clear in the literature that a calorie deficit is absolutely necessary to lose weight, it's also a fact that hitting specific macro targets can be an advantage when you're trying to preserve muscle mass and blunt your hunger.

The good news is that you don't have to master the macro-tracking part of the game to make progress. You just have to start where you are. If you've never even heard of macronutrients before and you have a good twenty-plus pounds to lose, then your starting place will be to eat a little less than you have been each day—in other words, reducing calories. Concentrate on mastering the bottom of the pyramid before you worry about controlling your macronutrient intake.

Let's keep moving up the pyramid. Next step—micronutrition. Micronutrients include vitamins and minerals that your body needs for optimum health. When your diet is lacking in whole, minimally processed foods, micronutrient deficiencies may occasionally cause issues. What you'll see, though, is that if you get your macronutrients and calorie intake managed it is unlikely that you'll have to worry too much about micronutrients. If you are small enough in stature to have a lower calorie intake for maintenance, or if you tend to eat a lot of crap (which people will often attempt as long as the crap in question "fits their macros") you may want to consider some vitamin and mineral supplementation. I think most people can get by just fine without supplements of any kind, but we'll take a closer look at them later.

Our second-to-highest pyramid level is meal timing. If you ask the average person which will make their metabolism burn faster, six smaller meals a day or three normal sized meals, nine out of ten* people will tell you that smaller meals is the answer. We'll explore this more in a later chapter, but let me say that for the most part, meal timing doesn't matter that much. So, if you've been packing six small meals a day and hauling all of that back and forth to work, you can relax about that. The trend of intermittent fasting is helping to change peoples' minds about many small meals in a day, but it sometimes seems like it takes one fad to replace another. We'll talk more about intermittent fasting later. But that does go to show that a big part of the problem when it comes to understanding the fundamentals is that there is so much misleading advice out there creating confusion for would-be dieters.

> *I made this statistic up, but after you read this book quiz the people you know—nearly everyone believes this.

And finally, the top of the pyramid: supplements. Keep in mind that as we go up the pyramid, we're going from the most important things to the least. For many people, supplements are totally unnecessary, especially any of the so-called "fat burners," which are primarily expensive caffeine pills. However, there are a few things worth taking for general health. We'll get into those details in a later chapter.

So, there you have it. The pyramid of dieting importance. Often, people get stuck in a "gathering information" mindset, but you don't have to master the entire pyramid to make major progress. It's your consistency over time that will move the needle of your scale down in a smart, sustainable way.

So, to get going with good dieting habits, let's talk about becoming "calorically aware."

FOUR
Tracking Your Calorie Intake

To start moving the needle on the scale the way we want it to go, we're going to borrow some time-tested techniques of bodybuilders. Don't worry. I'm not going to ask you to lube up and pose in a skimpy bikini or banana hammock in front of a large audience. But when it comes to dropping body fat, these guys and gals have it down to a science. And almost without exception, they use an organized system to track their caloric and macronutrient intake.

The idea here is to tackle the bottom of the pyramid first. Getting your overall food intake under control is the first step to getting you where you want to be. Without that, nothing else higher on the pyramid is going to matter that much.

So, don't even think about supplements until you get your intake under control. There are no magic pills!

It just makes sense. If you want to keep your bank balance on the right side of zero, you must track your spending. And if you want to fit into your skinny pants again, you're going to have to track your food intake. At least for a while. The more you become "calorie aware," the less you will have to track every little thing. But for now, we want to set goals for your daily intake, macronutrient intake (at least protein, but if you're new to this and want to make progress, track fats and carbohydrates too), and possibly alcohol intake if you happen to be a regular drinker. (More on the whole drinking thing later.)

There are several ways to track your food intake. But before you know what your goal is going to be, you need to know your basic calorie requirements. And you need to keep in mind that whatever you come up with is just a starting point. Remember, there is not a huge difference between individuals when it comes to how quickly calories are burned up, but some people tend to fidget more than others or have a higher "body thermostat" than average.

Pick an app for your phone to keep track of your calorie intake. There are many to choose from, so read up on them and pick whichever one resonates with you the most. You must commit to using the app religiously for the next month or maybe longer, but definitely not less than that. And when I say track your food with an app, what I mean is "weigh and measure every single bite you put into your mouth for one month." Weighing your food will show you where much of your diet problem might lie. For example, if you weigh a bowl of cereal, you might see that you've been eating three servings at a time instead of just one.

> Some of the more popular tracking apps are listed below. I'm personally a My Fitness Pal man, and it's the most popular of the choices listed.
> - My Fitness Pal
> - My Plate
> - Lose It!
> - Fooducate

Another benefit of tracking your intake is that you'll see which foods you like that are lower in calories than you ever realized. Once you find a few of those kinds of choices you can start eating more of those and less of the higher calorie items. Those little substitutions can go a long way to getting you to your goal.

What usually happens when people begin to track their food consumption accurately is that they start to avoid snacking. ("I'm not going to eat that so I don't have to whip my phone out and add it to my day, which is looking pretty good so far.") For many people, it becomes a game to eat foods with lower caloric density and keep their daily consumption under their desired amount.

Speaking of your daily intake amount, you may be wondering how much you should be aiming for when it comes to setting up your app. Good question. Let's talk about that now.

Most of the apps you might use to keep track of your food intake will use the well-known Mifflin-St. Jeor equation to determine your Basal Metabolic Rate (BMR). Your BMR is the calories you'd burn through if you sat on your couch and didn't move at all for 24 hours. To find the number of calories you need in a day, you should start with your BMR and add the calories required to move around, exercise, and do other life activities.

Many of the popular apps will give you an "estimated burn" for different activities. Please don't use them. It's hard enough to keep an accurate count of what you're eating day to day, let alone trying to deduct from that total an estimate of calories burned. It's simply too confusing.

➡ It's also the reason you'll use an "activity modifier" when figuring out your caloric needs. That modifier will take your exercise burn into account.

Now we can figure out maintenance calories, the calories you must eat to stay the same weight from day to day. The only reason we're going to add an activity multiplier to your BMR is to figure out what your maintenance calories are. Once we figure out your maintenance calories, we can figure out how much to cut from that number to start dropping some weight.

Below is the Basal Metabolic Rate equation for men and women. Note that these calculations determine your basal metabolic rate calories.

- **Men:** 10 × weight (kg) + 6.25 × height (cm) − 5 × age (years) + 5
- **Women:** 10 × weight (kg) + 6.25 × height (cm) − 5 × age (years) − 161

Now you'll have to add an activity multiplier to get your total maintenance calories:

- BMR × 1.200 = sedentary (little or no exercise)

- BMR × 1.375 = light activity (light exercise/sports 1–3 days/week)
- BMR × 1.550 = moderate activity (moderate exercise/sports 3–5 days/week)
- BMR × 1.725 = very active (hard exercise/sports 6–7 days a week)
- BMR × 1.900 = extra active (very hard exercise/sports and physical job)

Sorry for all the math. There are plenty of online calculators that will do the heavy lifting for you, and pretty much every app you could use to track your food consumption will perform these calculations too.

Now that you've calculated your BMR and added your activity multiplier, you need to determine how many calories to remove from what you just came up with to decide on your daily caloric deficit, meaning how many fewer calories you need to eat to start losing weight. Let's say you're going for a pound of fat loss a week. This is the most common scenario for those trying to drop 10–20 pounds.

A pound of fat is equal to about 3,500 calories. To lose that one pound of fat per week, you'll need to remove 500 calories per day from your intake. 500 calories isn't too harsh. You can remove those calories by avoiding some of the more "snacky" items from your daily menu and barely even notice the difference. And if you substitute some of the higher-density foods from your current staples for something with more fiber or protein, it's likely that you'll feel more full than usual while you're dropping pounds week after week.

> A pound of fat, by the way, is about the size of a large lemon. Start removing large lemons from your love handles, and it doesn't take long to make some big changes.

Every two to four weeks you'll start to notice your weight loss leveling off or slowing down. The reason is that if you've lost weight, there is now less of you. This smaller amount of you is now burning fewer calories overall, so you'll have to either a) increase your daily activity to burn more calories, or b) eat even less. At some point, you'll find that you're going to have to either be happy with where you are or push harder than before to improve. Simple, but not easy.

One very important thing to remember is this: all these calculations are only giving you an estimate. You are going to have to monitor your progress and see what works for you. If you are losing weight and maintaining muscle strength and bulk, you should keep on doing what you're doing. If you're following the recommendations of the BMR calculator but not seeing progress, you will need to make adjustments.

What isn't as simple as tracking your food intake is tracking your weight loss and knowing when things are truly stalled versus if you're just retaining water. Weight loss is never linear beyond the initial stage when you're dropping the first five pounds or so. You can expect some back and forth motion on the needle of your scale, but don't panic. As your fat cells empty, it is common to start retaining more water than usual, which might keep the scale from budging for days, sometimes weeks. Hold the course! Often the body will lose a lot of that water very quickly and you'll be five pounds lighter overnight. Sometimes more.

This phenomenon is known in bodybuilding circles as the "whoosh effect," and it happens more often in women. So if you're tracking your food intake and you know you're in a calorie deficit but the scale doesn't seem to be moving the way it should—be patient. Wait for the whoosh. Don't further restrict your calories until you've hit the next level. Too much restriction will make your life miserable before it's necessary.

The good news is that you can get lean and mean long before you get to the point where you're suffering. The people who suffer the most are looking to get ripped abs. That kind of extended dieting and super low body fat levels will make the body fight back to keep from starving. There's nothing wrong with six-pack abs, but you should know ahead of time that getting that lean essentially means going to war with your body's genetic programming to not starve to death.

> Let's be honest, dieting is never going to be comfortable. The trick is making it suck less while you're getting the best results.

If you're in the "I just need to drop 10–20 pounds" club a good general rule of thumb is to diet for weight loss (BMI plus activity multiplier minus daily caloric deficit) for four weeks at a time. Then you can take a one- to two-week break where you eat at your new maintenance calories (BMI plus activity multiplier). Then you can go back to your weight loss routine again. If your body spends too long a time in a caloric deficit, you'll find that your body will start to rebel against you by making you ravenously hungry.

Also, the longer you're in a calorie-deficit, the more your cortisol levels will rise. Higher cortisol means more hunger, less sleep, and a higher sense of being stressed out. So short breaks where you eat at your maintenance level of calories will reduce your mental and physical stress. Losing a pound a week throughout a year, even with these occasional diet breaks thrown in, you're still in the neighborhood of 50 pounds lost. And when you do it this way instead of following the extremes of the fad diet world, you'll be much more likely to keep the pounds off, which is the real challenge for most people. So, play the long game, and master these fundamentals.

FIVE
Flexibility Is the Key

And no, I don't mean being able to do the splits. People who have the most success with fat loss and body composition goals are all over the map when it comes to personality types. Some people are built for daily tracking and relish the idea of making a spreadsheet to fine-tune their math. Some people are on the opposite end of the spectrum, and the idea of logging every meal seems like more work than could ever be worth it. They would rather be fat than try.

Most people are somewhere in the middle, and their ability to pay attention to the details waxes and wanes with their schedules and daily life stresses. I get it. I go through seasons where I meticulously track every bite, only to follow it by months of skipping breakfast, eating a sandwich and a protein bar at lunch, and then pigging out at dinner hoping that I left enough caloric space at the end of the day to maintain my desired weight.

> Of course, I've been doing this for years and have a better intuition about it than most people.

Often the hardest part of fat loss is sticking to the plan when it seems like it's not working. What I'm getting at here is that you must be flexible, but still find ways to stay the course. There are times when the scale won't seem to be moving at all, and you'll want to quit and binge on pizza.

> Since fat loss is not linear, sometimes the best thing to do is to make no changes and give your body a chance to "catch up" with the calorie deficit.

Sometimes sticking to the program means that you need to assess your intake with a little more scrutiny. Sometimes, you need to relax about your "allowed" foods and give yourself a broader palate of foods from which to choose. A mindset of flexibility will tell you that you can have a couple of slices, but then go back and stick to your plan.

We all know it's true: weight maintenance is a lifestyle. So, you have to pick a diet that you can maintain. One that's based on your preferences, not just what the latest celebrity is doing this week. Often, the people who are hyper detail-oriented tend to classify foods into "good" and "bad" categories, and then avoid anything in the latter classification. Let me tell you that assigning a moral value to food is a bad idea.

Let's take sugar, for example. Many, if not most, people would say that sugar is terrible, but let's look at sugar consumption in context. Let's say that you are in your calorie deficit and your deficit number is 1,900 per day. And let's say that you've hit your protein intake for the day, have worked out with weights, and still have a couple of hundred calories left in your budget. So, you eat some ice cream. You have no aversion to dairy, you've eaten your share of veggies for the day and even had a little fruit to provide some of your carbs after your workout. Is that ice cream bad?

If you've hit your goals for the day and eaten enough whole, minimally refined or processed foods to get your micronutrients, I would propose that a little extra glucose is going to be good for your soul. A little ice cream reward at the end of a tough day will prevent you from binging on the full carton if you try to stick to some stringent, mythical perfect diet. And in my experience, the people who leave room in their daily intake for a little flexibility are the ones who can keep it going for the long haul. Besides, who wants to live in a world without ice cream?

What you need to do is write out a list of the foods that you prefer, and then do a quick check of their calories. Based on your findings, you can make menus for yourself that will keep everything in check ahead of time.

That way you will have a list of menus to choose from when time is at a premium. Also, your list will be composed of foods that you actually like. I can't tell you how many times I've had people tell me that they lost weight doing something like the keto diet for a few months, but then put it all back on and then some as soon as they left that restrictive way of eating.

You will fail in your quest to lose fat and then keep it off with too rigid a mindset. You must eat foods you like to have long-term success. Just not too much. So be flexible, eat the foods you like within reason, and enjoy the long-term success that comes from having the right mindset.

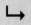 No lie, I often eat a bowl of cereal for a snack, but I use a protein drink for the milk.

SIX
Suggested Rate of Fat Loss

We've talked about how to start losing the fat. Now let's talk about how fast that process should work. The answer, of course, is "it depends." It depends on how much you have to lose. It depends on your food preferences. It depends on what deadline you may be looking at—is there an event you're preparing for, like a wedding or a class reunion? Are you doing this for health? Aesthetics? These things matter when it comes to people's motivations to make the change.

One pound of fat is equal to about 3,500 calories. And although the metabolism of the human body has a lot of variables, it's a good number to shoot for when it comes to figuring out how much of a deficit it takes to drop the fat. Really big people require a lot more calories per day than smaller people, so if you have a lot of weight to lose that also means you have a lot more wiggle room when it comes to calculating your calorie deficit.

There are limits, too. If you have a lot to lose, like 50 to 100 lbs. or more, then your weight loss goal should be a max of four pounds a week. And that's pushing it. Anything more and you'll be losing more than just fat, and you want to preserve your muscle mass at all costs, even if it means slowing the rate of total weight loss.

Many females eat only around 1,800 calories for maintenance, so for a smaller-frame dude or most females the idea of dropping more than 500 calories a day isn't in the cards. At some point, the average person is just unwilling to eat less than a certain amount of food. Food is more than just fuel. It's a part of our lives.

For most people, aiming for 1% of body weight per week is a good target, unless you are already really lean and looking for that last bit of fat loss that will reveal your abs. Then you're looking at closer to .5% a week or even less.

And just because you can lose fat a little faster than 1% of body weight per week doesn't mean you should. The more severely you cut your calories, the more deprived you will feel and the harder it will be to maintain the momentum of weight loss. So what if you could eat no carbs for a month and lose a bunch of weight (much of which would be water, by the way), if the second you eat some pretzels you gained it all back?

Another potential problem with losing too much too fast is the fact that your skin won't have time to adapt as quickly as you're losing the fat. This can leave you with a band of loose skin around your midsection that you don't want. That can even happen with leaner individuals too. Not that I'm against feeling hungry or doing more aggressive dieting. There's plenty of literature to support the idea that losing weight quickly isn't better or worse than taking your time. But in the interest of building good habits, it's probably better to take your time and be deliberate and mindful about the process.

Another benefit of taking your time and getting good at your weight loss process is the fact that the process that gets you to your goal is the same process that will keep you at that goal—in other words, your flexible dieting plan. As you get better at the process you can eventually get yourself dialed in so that you're always just a couple of weeks away from your baseline weight/look. You can lose that last little bit of weight quicker if you follow the weight loss routine you had previously set out for yourself.

Something else to consider when you're working through the dieting process is that weight loss is not a linear event. I keep saying that, because it's important. It takes consistency over time to get results. Often people jump from program to program looking for a quick fix, when they could have kept doing what they were doing for just a little while longer and gotten the best results.

Once you calculate the weight loss and maintenance routine that you will follow, you're getting to the real work of fat loss: learning to stay in the saddle day in and day out, eating from a list of meals that you've got down cold when it comes to tracking, possibly avoiding certain social settings to achieve your goals, making the small sacrifices it takes to keep moving the needle on your scale and doing it on autopilot as much as possible so you don't wear yourself out mentally.

Hitting a plateau is often very upsetting for people who haven't yet hit their fat loss goal, but I'd like to suggest that holding at that plateau for a few weeks is an excellent way to practice maintaining your new weight. Maintaining weight loss is far harder than achieving it in the first place, but when you look at a plateau as merely practice at holding your new lower weight it can be liberating. It should be a minor victory to hold onto to this new "progress weight" for a few weeks before further weight loss kicks in. After all, the ultimate goal is to coast into that particular plateau that also happens to be your end goal.

> Although, the beauty of the flexible approach is that you can more easily navigate social situations without worrying about "messing up your diet." You just eat a little less earlier in the day so you have a little more wiggle room later. More on this later when we get to meal timing.

It's essential to the process that you get to your goal in a way you don't hate. Because getting there while hating the process is an excellent way to hit your target and then revert right back to the behavior that caused the weight gain in the first place. You don't want that, but it's very likely that it's already happened in your dieting history. And if it has, the next chapter is for you.

SEVEN
Goals Versus Habits

Over the years my philosophy has changed regarding the title of this chapter. I've had many conversations with people who have lost a lot of weight, and even more importantly, kept it off. Without fail the "secret sauce" proves to be their daily habits when it comes to diet and exercise.

Let's think this through. Habits are systems for getting results. Goals are what you want the results to be. Goals are the imaginary endpoint where one will finally achieve happiness, and habit systems are the day-to-day grind one has to embrace to make progress toward those goals.

One of the most essential traits of anyone who has achieved and maintained their weight loss goals is that they have learned to embrace the journey. They have daily rituals, or habits, that keep them on track. For many, those rituals include things such as tracking their intake, prepping a bunch of meals for the upcoming week, getting up at a particular time every day to exercise, and going to bed at the same time every night to ensure adequate sleep.

You need a system to guide your daily behavior in a way that will slowly but surely get you to your weight goal even if your goal changes, as goals often do, which is completely normal. When you focus on creating the routine that will support the physical changes you want to achieve, you will start making those important daily wins that eventually stack the bricks into a new house, or a new body. And sometimes, in diet land, that means embracing not just routine, but boredom.

Variety of food is a good thing, but it can also lead to overeating. Consider your behavior when going to a buffet, or on Thanksgiving with the family. The more choices, the higher the pile on your plate will be. A good strategy is to embrace boredom for your lunch every day, not battle it. Eat something you've pre-prepped for the week and can account for easily on your tracking sheet or app. I've been doing this for years minus the occasional business lunch. On those occasions, I aim for some higher protein fare and try not to get too clenched up about it.

And it's easy for me not to get clenched up about it, because almost every day I stick with the program and eat my boring lunch, go to the gym, and read for a few minutes before returning to my office. Embracing a boring lunch also helps me have a much less boring dinner, which is the meal I'm likely to eat with my family and will want to eat a little more than one serving. Lunch is just fuel to finish my work day. Dinner is fuel for my soul. So, a boring lunch is okay.

Now, you don't have to pick daily lunches as your boring meal. You may love lunch. You don't have to have any boring meals at all. The point is, eating the same thing for lunch every day is a habit I and many other fitness professionals embrace to maintain our body fat levels. If you find a few go-to meals that meet your calorie and nutritional requirements and eat them every day you will start dropping fat on autopilot.

Now let's talk about the downside of goals.

First off—nobody knows what kind of goals they should stick with. We think we want to drop x amount of body fat, or fit back into our wedding dress, or look awesome at our class reunion. What we don't often realize is that as we move toward our goal, it will start to change.

For instance, say someone has the goal of getting six-pack abs. Many dudes have this goal because they think when they get those abs they will have happiness in their lives and the woman of their dreams will fall into their arms. So they implement some habits that start getting them leaner. They hit the gym. They mind their caloric intake and aim to hit their protein target for the day. They don't screw it up on the weekends (which is a big mistake people make).

Weeks become months, and our hero starts to see the blurry outline of his rectus abdominis in the mirror. But...

He's also begun to look smaller in the mirror, especially in the chest and arms. And what's worse is that people are always asking him if he's okay, saying he looks unhealthy or sick, even.

Our hero then decides to put some weight back on his frame. Now he is five pounds higher than six-pack weight, and the comments go from "you look sick," to "you've lost some weight!" which is code for "you're looking good."

Should our hero regret all the progress he's made because he didn't reach his goal of being six-pack lean? No! He has changed his blood lipids for the better, is lighter on his feet, and has finally found the important balance between aesthetics and performance as he progressed through his journey.

I should know. That guy is me.

When I get truly ripped, my face looks too gaunt. My eyes get that sunken-in look that makes me look like I just escaped from prison. If I get lean enough to have six-pack abs, the bones of my pelvis jut out with no padding, which really sucks when I graze the kitchen counter by accident. So, I stay slightly less lean than that and have found that I stay plenty satisfied with my appearance anyway.

There are other downsides to focusing too rigidly on goals. A major one is delaying gratification until you hit your goal. What that means is telling yourself "I'll be happy when I get there." And then when you do get there—what next? Achieving a goal is a good reason to celebrate, but the achievement comes and goes quickly. And often, achieving a goal kills the motivation.

I know several people who have competed in marathons. They trained hard, ate right, and finished the race—and then immediately piled back on the weight they had lost during their training, and even more. One guy did this several times over the years and eventually ended up having bariatric surgery to force himself to eat less because he would balloon up so fast after a race.

Everyone's goal is to at least finish the race, metaphorically speaking. Not everyone does. But we tend to concentrate on the ones who do. In other words, we believe the ones who achieve their goal are the happiest. However, the ones who improve their level of fitness simply by preparing for the dietary race are often the happiest regardless of what place they came in at the finish line, or if they finished at all.

What I'm getting at here is that goal-oriented thinking often leads to the situation where our happiness depends upon achieving that single goal. Instead, we should focus more on the routine habits that support our continued improvements as we move through life.

EIGHT
The Second Step of the Pyramid: Macros

To review: overall caloric intake is the most important factor when losing weight. That's why calories make the broad base of our pyramid. However, there are some tweaks you can make to your macronutrient intake that will make it much easier to keep your total calories down while retaining muscle, if you're exercising.

As I said at the beginning of this book, exercise isn't great for creating a calorie deficit. But it is fantastic at building and retaining muscle while you are on a diet. So, to lose fat instead of muscle, you should exercise AND get plenty of the first macro we're going to discuss: protein.

Protein: Your Ally in the Battle of the Bulge

Ahh, protein. How I love you for your ability to satisfy my appetite, build and maintain muscle, and make this dieting thing a whole lot easier.

Protein is composed of amino acids and when eaten, broken back down into them by your digestive system. Your muscles, skin and hair, tendons and ligaments, and all kinds of cellular machinery are composed of protein.

There are 21 total amino acids that the body needs. Out of that 21, your body can manufacture only twelve of them. The other nine are essential, meaning we must supply them by eating foods that contain those amino acids. One of the reasons we consume protein is to get the essential amino acids our bodies can't manufacture so that our bodies can repair and restore the tissues that we wear out by merely existing.

And some people do a lot more than exist. They exercise or have physically demanding jobs. Those are the people who have an increased need for protein intake. But there are others whose need is not so obvious: anyone who is dieting.

Since muscle is built from protein, you need to keep feeding your muscles the right amino acids during your diet to keep them from being whittled away while you're losing weight. Muscles are metabolically expensive to maintain as it is, but if you don't feed them the raw materials necessary for their preservation, you'll start losing them right along with the fat. So if you're dieting and not preserving muscle mass, you're going to be working your way to the "skinny fat" look that nobody wants.

You also need to send your body the signal to maintain muscle retention and growth: exercise. Pick your poison, but know that strength training will be the strongest signal to your body that your muscles are essential and need to hang around for the after-diet party.

There are many potential sources of protein. The first things that come to mind with most people are animal products and dairy. And indeed, these are excellent choices for bumping up your protein intake, as they generally have much more complete amino acid profiles. Everything you need to preserve your muscle mass can be found in meat, fish, eggs, and milk.

One common objection to eating a high-protein diet is the fear of damage to the kidneys. These fears are unfounded—there has been no study to date that has found that higher protein intake damages healthy kidneys. If you have compromised kidney function you should work with a registered dietician who has experience with setting up diets for those in that situation.

Another legitimate concern with a high-protein diet is the fact that higher protein often means a higher intake of saturated fats. Higher saturated fat intake is associated with elevated LDL cholesterol levels, which are associated with elevated risk of heart disease.

You don't want to get ripped and pretty just to punch out early because you had a fatal heart attack.

Thus, the emphasis is on leaner cuts of meat. I know. This is as hard for me to write as it is for you to read. And I admit to having my share of fatty steaks and pot roasts and beef ribs and such. After all, I'm writing this from Houston, Texas. In Texas, the four food groups are chili, barbeque, fajitas, and steaks. You could say we're at the top of our class for saturated fat intake. But lower saturated fat intake is important for a high-protein diet.

> It's also really hard to track the fat content of fattier cuts of meat, so your caloric intake can get away from you quickly if you eat too much of it.

It can be a challenge to keep your saturated fat intake lower on a diet high in animal products, so you should keep an eye out for leaner cuts. I normally recommend choosing the leaner cuts of meat (although I do love a good ribeye on occasion), but I tend to choose a higher fat content with dairy because I can't stand the taste of low-fat dairy products. (But if you can then it might be a good idea to select low-fat dairy products as well.)

The good news is that eating more vegetables can help mitigate the effects of eating more saturated fats, to a degree. A higher vegetable intake also means more fiber, more micronutrients, and a higher food volume at a lower caloric cost. That means if you eat more veggies, it will protect you somewhat from some of the negatives associated with higher meat consumption while simultaneously helping you eat less overall, since vegetables fill you up faster and keep you feeling full longer, just like protein but for different reasons.

Another way to take a half step farther up our pyramid of diet importance is to aim for a specific amount of protein every day but not track other macros. For most people, this technique will prevent overeating even without tracking carbs and fat, because protein is so satisfying that you will automatically eat less. Ironically, many people who have a hard time sticking to a specific calorie target will have a hard time eating enough when really going for it with the protein. Research shows that eating a high-protein diet can cause an automatic decrease in overall calorie consumption. A paper published in the National Center for Biotechnology Information states that "A high-protein diet induces sustained reductions in appetite, ad libitum caloric intake, and body weight." The authors concluded that "An increase in dietary protein from 15% to 30% of energy at a constant carbohydrate intake produces a sustained decrease in ad libitum caloric intake...This anorexic effect of protein may contribute to the weight loss produced by low-carbohydrate diets" (Weigle, Breen, et al).

So in laymen's terms, eating more protein makes you eat less of the other stuff, and the increase in daily protein that happens with low-carb diets is probably why low-carb diets work. It's not the lower carbs causing the effect, it's the high protein intake blunting your appetite for more calories.

Setting your protein intake target depends on your gender and on the percent of body fat you have. If you are a male and have 20% body fat or less, or a female and have less than 35% body fat, aim for one gram of protein per pound of body weight per day. So if you are a dude who weighs 175 pounds, eat 175 grams of protein every day. You will be feeling very full, my friend. You will preserve muscle, and maybe even build some more if your gym routine is strong.

How do you measure how much body fat you have? Calculating body fat percentage can be tricky. Those scales that supposedly tell you by using electrical impedance through your hands or feet? Completely and horribly inaccurate. But there are several ways to measure yourself at home, the most popular of which involves a pair of calipers.

Calipers are only as good as the person using them, and they are hard to use on yourself. If you belong to a gym, there will usually be a trainer who's done many such measurements. This is your go-to person. Even easier, and maybe better, is to Google "body fat percentage pictures" and compare yourself to what you see there. For the most part, though, you probably intuitively know if you are overweight or just have a little extra chunk to whittle off.

If you figure out that you are over the recommended body fat percentage for the "gram per pound" formula above, there are two other ways to configure your protein needs: You could set your daily protein intake at 40% of your total daily calorie intake, which should be fairly easy for you to calculate. The 40% thing is something you can do with almost every tracking app out there. Or, you can set it for one gram of protein per pound of your desired body weight. An example of the desired body weight equation looks like this: a female who weighs 180 pounds who wants to weigh 130 would set her protein intake at 130 grams per day. Easy.

Increased protein intake is one of your best friends for losing body fat while escaping the "skinny fat" look that is common when people jump on the fad diet train without learning the truth about what they need to eat and why, when it comes to retaining muscle mass. But there's another ally in the muscle-preserving battle that you must fight in the war against skinny fatness: carbohydrates. We'll talk about them next.

Carbohydrates: Friend or Enemy?

No other macronutrient fills people with fear these days like carbs. But just so we're all on the same page about what a carb actually is, let's run through the basics.

Carbohydrates are sugar molecules of different lengths. There are simple and complex carbs, and as you might imagine, the simple ones are the shorter chains, while complex carbs are composed of longer chains.

There are three different chain categories: monosaccharides, oligosaccharides, and polysaccharides. Mono means one, and monos are the simplest of the three—when you eat monos they can't be broken down any further since they are already in their purest form. The oligosaccharides are short chains of monos. Sucrose, otherwise known as table sugar, is an example of an oligosaccharide. Polysaccharides or complex carbs are long chains of monos.

Complex carbs take longer for your body to break down, have more fiber, and are considered healthier in general. They should be your mainstay carb sources. Examples would be oats, rice, whole grains, vegetables, and fruits.

Polysaccharides can be further classified by their digestibility: digestible, partially digestible, and indigestible. Starches like you find in potatoes are an example of a digestible (and delicious) polysaccharide. Beans have quite a bit of the partially digestible kind of polys, which means your body doesn't actually do the work of digesting them but the gas-causing bacteria in your gut does, which is why beans are the musical fruit. An example of the indigestible polys would be cellulose—think corn.

Most of the carbs we eat have some protein or fat in them, too. Beans, for instance, have some protein and some starch along with the music-inducing partially digestible polysaccharides. Carb-rich foods can also have more than one kind saccharide, too.

One of the most irritating things about the current low-carb craze is that people are actively avoiding fruit consumption, which is a great way to deprive themselves of essential micronutrients and fiber. Fruit tends to be low calorie, too. Try replacing your daily candy bar with an apple and the needle will start to move on the scale with just that one substitution.

There is a place for the simple, quick digesting carbs, too—just before or after a workout when your body needs the fuel and is primed to store it efficiently. A handful of sugary candy 30 minutes before lifting weights or running can give you a little extra push.

Carbs are also the preferred source of fuel for your brain and nervous system. Your brain consumes about 120 grams of glucose a day. That's right—your brain uses about 480 calories of glucose a day.

As usual, it's all about context. Hard-line low-carbers will say there's no reason to eat simple sugars ever, but avoiding the fuel source your muscles prefer for contractions that are involved in activities like lifting weights or sprinting is self-sabotage.

Often, people who go on a very low-carb diet (keto) report a two-week or so period of "brain fog" as they enter the state of ketosis. Ketosis means that your body is releasing ketones into the system. Ketones are chemicals made in the liver from fat your body uses for energy when there's no glucose in the house, and "brain fog" refers to a mild intermittent state of confusion which may occur when your body is working hard to switch over from breaking down glucose to breaking down your body fat. Your brain can use ketones, but there's a difference between merely "being able" to do something, and "optimal." Since using glucose is your brain's default setting, it's far more likely that glucose is optimal for the brain.

Glucose is also optimal for muscular performance. There are occasional exceptions, but so far no professional sports team, no matter what the sport, has switched their players to a very low-carb diet. The players need the fuel that glucose provides.

One pervasive idea in the world of fad diets is the idea that carbs, and by extension insulin, are responsible for the increased girth seen across the land. The general thinking goes like this: Carb consumption triggers the secretion of insulin. Insulin is a storage hormone that assists in placing these sugars into muscle tissue. Insulin also prevents body fat from being used as a fuel source. Therefore, a diet that promotes circulating insulin (i.e., promotes normal consumption of carbs) is believed to lead to weight gain.

Several diet fads push the idea that the removal of carbs will enable the body to burn fat stores more easily, since carbs (and insulin) are what prevents the body from dipping into those stores. Insulin, they say, is the enemy. It must be minimized.

Of course, it's not so simple. It never is. But in this case we don't want it to be simple, because carbs are delicious and we want to eat them if we can. To that end, let's take a closer look at insulin—what it does and doesn't do, and why it may just be the most misunderstood hormone of all.

Let's tackle the biggest fear people have about insulin first: that insulin causes fat storage. While this is true, it's also the case that fat can be stored without insulin. An enzyme known as Hormone Sensitive Lipase can cause fat storage even when the level of circulating insulin is low. If your calorie intake is too high, regardless of the kind of food that makes up those calories, fat storage is going to happen regardless of an insulin response.

Another common myth about insulin is that carbs are the sole stimulator of this hormone. This isn't true. Protein-rich foods will have the same effect as carbs and, as we've seen, protein is your friend in the battle of the bulge. People often assume that insulin release increases hunger as well, but the fact is that insulin blunts hunger. The insulin response to a meal is one of the reasons you start feeling full and stop eating.

Eating a little carbohydrate will usually only raise insulin (in healthy individuals) for a given time after a meal, not all day long. It goes like this: you eat, glucose enters your bloodstream, insulin rises to deal with it, everything is stored to the muscles, the liver, or in fat cells (usually all three), then your glucose level drops, and insulin levels drop too. Wash, rinse, repeat this cycle all day long. When insulin is done with its job, your body goes back to fat burning. If you're keeping your total daily calorie allotment under what you normally use, when the insulin level goes back down you will go back to using the energy stored in your fat cells to take up the slack. If you also keep your protein intake relatively high and do resistance exercises, you will do a much better job of losing fat.

So—it's not the insulin response to eating carbs that has given carbs a bad rep. But still, you say, low-carb diets really seem to work for many people. Why are they working so well? Why do low-carb diets seem to trend every few years?

Well, one reason is that a misunderstanding of what we discussed above seems to pop up every so often. But that doesn't explain why people have success with low-carb diets. It's that initial success that perpetuates the myths about insulin, and round and round we go.

The success of low-carb diets comes down to the fact that when you're avoiding an entire macronutrient, it is going to be a whole lot harder for you to overeat. Eating less means you'll be burning more calories than you're consuming. Also, eating fewer carbs means you'll be eating a little more of something else, and that something else is often protein which, as we've discussed, is awesome for many reasons when it comes to dropping body fat.

I have no problem with lower carb diets, by the way. It's just the misunderstanding about how they work that I find irritating. And I should mention that I used to believe the above myths myself, so no judgment here. But knowing the truth can set you free.

And the truth is, most of the foods that people think of when they think of "carbs" are foods like donuts, crackers, chips, and other calorie-dense, high-fat, high-carb foods. But a food that is as high in fat as it is in carbs is not just a carb. It's a mix, and it just so happens to be a mix of macros that most people find irresistible. For many, the super-delicious mix of carbs and fats is the primary cause of their weight gain over the years. And I don't know about you, but I can eat a lot of French fries in one sitting. Add up a few sittings a week, and you can see where that will get you.

Furthermore, the fat/carb combo can be insidiously tricky to track. Take crackers, for instance—some brands have more fat than others, and serving size makes a huge difference. Recently I compared some pretzel sticks to some popular brand-name crackers we had in our pantry. It took 26 pretzel sticks to equal the caloric density of five crackers. I can eat five crackers in about thirty seconds. The low-fat pretzel sticks slow me down a lot more. Since they're low fat, I quickly get tired of eating them and therefore am less likely to overindulge. That's my personal preference, though. It may not be yours. But one of the keys to getting and staying lean is finding small substitutions for higher-calorie snacks, so they don't do so much damage when you visit the pantry after hours.

That being said, many people seem to thrive on low-carb diets. My general advice when considering low-carb diets depends on your level of activity and how much body fat you need to lose. The more body fat you have to carve off, the more likely it is that your body doesn't need the carb-based fuel for activity. Let it use the fat stores instead.

If there is a lot of body fat present, it is also more likely that your ability to process glucose is somewhat impaired. The more overweight someone is, the more probable it is that they have insulin sensitivity issues. As the amount of stored body fat goes up, the body often becomes what's known as "insulin resistant," which means your pancreas keeps pumping out more insulin to store all the glucose and amino acids that keep coming on the scene.

The BMI, or body mass index, is a simple calculation that measures your body composition based on your height and weight. It's not perfect, but it's a good starting point to get a feel for where you are and how much you need to lose to start improving your essential health. Getting an accurate body fat percentage is tough, especially when you have larger fat stores, so if your score on the BMI is inching toward obese, then you can assume that you have some level of insulin resistance. Specific blood tests can determine if you have a sensitivity to insulin but as a rule of thumb, if you're a man and over, say, 20% body fat, it's likely you have some insulin resistance. For women, that percentage is closer to 30%.

So, if you're sedentary and don't need much fuel, or if you're insulin resistant, a low-carb approach would make sense in the early days of your weight loss journey. The good news is this: as you get leaner your ability to process and use carbs comes back online as your insulin resistance goes down. There's even a nice little "carb hack" you can use when you're lean that can potentially help reset a hunger hormone in your favor so that you can stay lean more easily.

We'll talk about that later in the book, but for now, know that if you're in the population who will have success with lower carbs, the avoidance of carbs isn't a life sentence.

Dietary Fat—Tastes Great, Easy to Overeat

Like carbohydrates, fats come in different forms. So let's talk about them.

Fats are organic molecules composed of chains of carbon and hydrogen molecules. There are three general types of fats: saturated, monounsaturated, and polyunsaturated. The three labels refer to the "saturation" or number of hydrogen atoms attached to the carbon backbone.

A molecule of saturated fat has no place where a hydrogen atom isn't attached. Saturated fats are usually solid at room temperature. The two most common sources of saturated fat are animal fats and tropical oils such as coconut oil.

Monounsaturated fats have one carbon in the chain that is "double bonded" to another because there is a missing hydrogen atom. This causes a small kink in the carbon chain and makes it so that the monos are liquid at room temperature. Examples of monounsaturated fats are avocado oil, olive oil, and seed oils.

Polyunsaturated fats have more than one double bond or kink in the molecule (poly=more than one) and are missing at least two hydrogen atoms. Examples are fish oil and flax oil.

I should also mention trans fats here. Trans fats are man-made fats for the most part although there are some naturally occurring trans fats (but they don't have the same negative health implications). They are used primarily to make baked goods last longer and other foods taste better. Trans fats are supposed to enhance "mouth feel," which just sounds gross. Trans fats are made by taking unsaturated fats and bubbling hydrogen through them to supply the missing hydrogen atoms in the molecules to create a saturated fat that will become solid at room temperature.

And trans fats are terrible for you. Your body doesn't know what to do with them. They harden the arteries and the cellular membranes. They contribute to all kinds of health issues, from Alzheimer's, to cholesterol imbalances, and heart disease. Fortunately, the market is responding to the demand to have them removed from some of the foods you eat so there are fewer of them to avoid now, but they're still out there. Look for the word "hydrogenated" on the label when you are in doubt. Hydrogenation is the process by which other fats become bad, man-made trans fats.

Just don't eat them. Okay? Okay.

Now that we know the basics, let's get into having the other types of fats in our diets.

The design of the human body requires a combination of all of these fats (except man-made trans fats). Monounsaturated fats are a mainstay of the Mediterranean diet, which has proven health benefits. I make a habit out of getting most of my daily fat quota from the monos. Olive oil is full of monos, and my go-to fat for cooking and for salad dressings and such. I'm also a huge fan of guacamole, which is made from avocados. Avocados and olive oil also contain polyunsaturated fats, which makes them mixed fat, but avocados and olive oil contain high levels of the monos.

> One tip that people often overlook is to weigh/measure the oil you use when cooking. Most people use the eyeball method when coating a pan to sauté something, and end up using more than three times

the amount they think they did. At 9 calories per gram, a few extra table-spoons here and there adds up quickly.

Polyunsaturated fatty acids (PUFAs) are what you get when you eat cold-water fish or take a fish oil supplement (one of the few supplements I recommend, by the way). But most of the oils consumed by Americans are omega-6 PUFAs derived from soybeans. PUFAs are also known as omega fatty acids. There are several types of omega fatty acids. The first type is omega-6 fatty acids, which are found in seeds and plants. There are also omega-3 fatty acids, which are the fish and flax oils mentioned above, and omega-9's which are found mainly in olive and avocado oils.

In a perfect world, we would be eating our share of omega-6s and 3s in a relatively even ratio. However, the current state of the American diet has us eating far more 6s than 3s by about a 16:1 ratio. The downside to getting that ratio out of balance is an increase in systemic inflammation which can lead to increased physical pain and higher susceptibility to different types of cancer.

One of the fastest ways to change your ratio of omega fatty acids is to lower your omega-6 intake by eating less fast food and fried food. You can also increase your omega-3 intake by eating more cold-water fish such as salmon or herring, or by taking a fish oil supplement.

The bottom line on fats, though, is this: they're easy for your body to store in excess, but you need a certain amount for cellular function, heart health, eye health, vitamin absorption, and even mental health. You should aim for at least 20% of your total daily calories to come from fats. Try to eat more healthy, monounsaturated fats and omega-3 polyunsaturated fats. Finally, try to limit your intake of saturated fats and omega-6 polyunsaturated fats, which is pretty easy to do if you simply eat less processed fast foods and fried foods.

Alcohol: The Fourth Macro

Alcohol is in its own category or macro because your body considers it to be poison. Because of that fact, when you drink alcohol, it goes straight to the top of your system's priorities when it comes to metabolizing it and getting it out of your body. Alcohol is seven calories per gram, making it a little less calorically dense than fat and slightly higher than protein or carbs. But what you probably really want to know is if you can drink and still lose fat.

The simple answer is: yes. The more honest answer, though, is: it depends.

> ⮕ You should just accept it right now: any amount of drinking while dieting is less than optimal. I'm not telling you what to do, but you've got to own this fact and prioritize appropriately.

It depends on your frequency of consumption, what type of booze you choose, and what happens to your willpower when it comes to snacking when you drink. And it's that last part that often causes a big struggle for people trying to lose fat while drinking.

When you drink alcohol, it converts to acetate in your liver and must be metabolized before anything else you eat, because your body has no storage mechanism for liquor but must get rid of it right away. And here's where the plot thickens. Studies (as well as practical experience) shows that nothing drives a person to eat a big, greasy meal at two in the morning like too much drinking. And the food you eat, especially the fatty foods you crave when you've been drinking, must somehow be stored while all that alcohol processing is going on. So fat storage is more likely to happen when you're imbibing, and there is also going to be a shutdown of fat burning during that time. When you drink, you're not burning fat, and you're storing everything you eat so your body can get to the booze processing first. None of that is going to help your fat loss goal.

But wait, there's more. Alcohol doesn't just throw off your groove with fat loss and storage, it also hampers muscle protein synthesis (MPS), which is the process by which you build more muscle.

Studies that have looked at the MPS and alcohol equation show that you'd have to be drinking quite a bit to screw up your gym gains. However, some people drink way more than they should. I can also tell you this—the easiest time I ever had to get really lean was when I abstained entirely from alcohol for *one full year*.

A little background—I knew I needed to slow down my alcohol consumption, but I was having a problem finding the sweet spot with moderation. I decided to take a full break from alcohol for one year. I wanted to see how I would feel, how I would sleep, and whatever else might happen.

Like I've said elsewhere in this book, our lives are largely a collection of our daily habits. Once I got my daily habit of not drinking going by finding substitutes for drinking behavior like making fancy-pants tea at night and drinking more mineral water for the taste of the fizz, it took no time to get into the groove.

One thing I loved about ditching the booze was that I could get away with a little more snacking at the end of the night and still maintain a decent calorie deficit. I started looking forward to my late-night crunch and better sleep a lot more than I cared about the two or three drinks I used to have every night.

I also got out of the groove of checking the scale all that often, but I noticed that my pants were getting looser. When I did take a peek at my weight one day I was shocked, for two different reasons. For one, I had gotten down to what I thought was my goal weight. But I was also shocked at how far I still needed to go to get the look I wanted. But I was able to get there in a year by staying on the wagon and doing many of the other things mentioned in this book.

If you choose to imbibe, one other thing to consider is the type of beverage you select. Beer is very calorically dense compared to most anything else (sorry, craft beer lovers—I feel your pain). Wine is next on the caloric density continuum. Finally, spirits like bourbon or vodka are on the low end.

What you mix with your drink can also have a dramatic impact on your overall calorie load, too. It's a good idea to play around with your tracking app and figure out what mixes and foods will do the least amount of damage ahead of time. Because, let's be honest—nobody is tracking their drinks in real time. It's best to have a plan in place before you leave for your night out.

The bottom line here is this—if you're focused on fat loss, you might want to consider taking a break from the bottle, or at least try cutting back. Just like when tracking your food, you should track how much you drink, because it'll be useful for your general understanding of where things might be going wrong.

NINE
Up the Pyramid: Meal Frequency

Pop quiz: which is more likely to increase your metabolic rate, six small meals a day or two much larger ones? I routinely ask people this question, and almost without fail people answer with six small meals. Many people I consult with often tell me they're struggling with their diet because of all the food prep they have to do and plastic containers they're hauling to work so they can keep "stoking the metabolic fires" all day long.

Here's the good news for almost anyone reading this: it doesn't really matter. And in my opinion, having two large meals that you look forward to is way more helpful psychologically than parsing out six snacks throughout the day that wouldn't satisfy a baby bird.

Since intermittent fasting is currently The Next Big Thing for many of the Hollywood elite and some of the bros at the gym, we need to talk about what it is, what it isn't, and how you can use meal frequency and timing as a tool to help you lose fat.

Let's start with the basics. Intermittent Fasting (IF) is a strategy for reducing your overall caloric intake by skipping a specified period of eating.

There are several popular methods of IF including Alternate Day Fasting (ADF) of various types as well as the popular Leangains method promoted by fitness professional Martin Berkhan. (He published a book about it in 2018, and if you go to leangains.com you can read his protocol in detail.)

ADF means that there will be days of the week where you fast by either not eating at all or eating many fewer calories than usual, often around 500 calories for the entire day. With ADF you fast at least once a week, but some people fast as frequently as every other day.

The Leangains method is set up using a 16:8 ratio. That means for 16 hours you fast, and your eating window is eight hours long. For most people, this can mean just skipping breakfast. Proponents say that using IF can trick your body into giving you all the benefits of calorie restriction while allowing you to eat pretty much whatever you want, but only during your eating window.

There is also a lot of talk on the internet about how IF has substantial health benefits by ramping up a process known as "autophagy" or cellular cleanup, meaning when the body clears out its dead and damaged cells. Unfortunately, the evidence isn't super strong that there are many health benefits to IF along those lines. And I wish there were, because I've followed the Leangains protocol for years now. The reason why I have done so is that despite the lack of unequivocal evidence for health improvement, I and many others have found that IF is an incredible tool when it comes to managing our overall calorie intake.

Here's why. I'm hard-wired not to be very hungry when I first wake up. And fortunately, despite the old saying, breakfast is not in fact the most important meal of the day. It's just one meal. But it happens to be a meal where people tend to eat the most calorie-dense yet nutritionally empty foods in existence, such as donuts, packaged cereal, waffles, and similar items.

Now don't get me wrong. I love those foods and occasionally have them, so no judgment here. But when you are trying to maintain a calorie deficit you have to pick your battles wisely. On a budget of 1,800 calories a day, eating 1,000 calories worth of fat and carbs in eight bites is unwise.

How I work it is: I drink coffee in the morning and go to work. I stay busy all morning and don't break for lunch until one o'clock. That's when I eat my first meal of the day, just before going to the gym (on the days that I do that). Since I'm not a big dude I have a relatively low caloric budget so my first meal tends to be small, with higher protein. I like to save most of my appetite for dinner at the end of my workday, which ends around six in the evening.

But oh, that evening meal is glorious. Because by now, I've worked all day, probably worked out at the gym, and now that the day is done I'm hungry. Since I've saved most of my calories for the end of the day I can eat a large meal and maybe even get seconds, and still be within my caloric budget. I can go to bed with a full belly.

Sometimes after dinner, I'll even have a little snack, maybe some popcorn or Greek yogurt with blueberries. But for the most part I try to let my dinner be my final meal of the day. I've been tracking my food long enough to where I know when I'm in the sweet spot of losing weight or if I'm going too far into the pantry. For me, one snack night on weekdays doesn't do any harm on the scale, but daily snacking does.

And that's how many people use IF. Not as a fad or "one weird trick" to burn belly fat but simply as a tool to manage calorie intake.

> If you ever see an article that starts with the title, "One Weird Trick," save yourself the trouble of reading it. There's no such thing.

There are some other benefits to fasting. First off, fasting helps you learn to distinguish hunger from boredom. It's easy to alleviate your boredom by popping something, anything, into your mouth. Second, fasting also helps you develop the necessary dietary self-control.

One idea you must embrace when you want to lose weight is the fact that you will have to deal with some low-grade hunger on occasion. Fasting helps you face that enemy on your terms, and once you get used to it you'll learn that the enemy has no teeth. In the past it would have been hard for me to fight the temptation to eat a piece or two or three of chocolate once I "broke the seal" on the day by eating breakfast. When I'm in my fasting mode, though, I can walk right past a bowl of chocolates because I'm not eating anything at all at that time. Skipping breakfast becomes no big deal if you can keep yourself busy and productive during the day.

For many people, the simple act of tracking their food intake trains their calorie awareness, but actually not eating for a certain set period during the day can show how often they were absent-mindedly snacking here and there. Once you remove those several hundred calories a day from "nibbles" you might find that the scale starts giving you more good news than bad without having to change much else.

Like I said, IF is a tool, but it's not one everyone should use. If you're pregnant, for instance, you should probably stick to a more regular meal frequency. If you have a history of suffering from an eating disorder you may want to skip this method. And some people find that they become hypoglycemic and tend to crash without some morning calories. But if you're feeling empowered by hearing that breakfast is not really the most important meal of the day, especially if you've always just kind of choked it down because you felt you should, you may want to consider the above approach to fasting.

TEN
Supplements: Don't Believe the Hype

I can't write an entire book about avoiding fad diets without discussing supplements. For the most part, supplements don't work for anything other than removing money from your wallet, with a few exceptions which we'll talk about in a minute. What I want to do right now is to try and talk you out of some of the recent fads in supplementation.

Number one on the hit parade: exogenous ketones.

If you've never heard of exogenous ketones (EK), let me catch you up to speed. Ketones are an alternate fuel source your body will make when there's not enough glucose for energy. Glucose, though, is the preferred source for both brain and muscle, as I've mentioned. But since "going keto" is all the rage right now, it was only a matter of time before a multi-level marketing company pumped out a product that would supposedly give you the benefits of going keto without having to do all that pesky dietary restriction.

The marketing literature used by such companies is full of how it could work, paired nicely with lots of testimonials and before/after pictures of people hyping the products. But there have been few studies showing real-world results. One of the more recent ones, published in 2017, revealed a disadvantage to cyclists using a ketone supplement. In fact, the study's title is: "Ketone diester ingestion impairs time-trial performance in professional cyclists." The key word here is "impairs."

In other words, save your money.

Next up on the list of supplements that don't do anything are the supposed "fat burners." Don't believe the hype that taking the latest fat-burning supplement will get you shredded. It might make you feel like a meth-head on a bender for an hour, but it isn't magically going to create the calorie deficit you need to lose your body fat. And almost without fail, the main ingredient in fat-burning supplements is caffeine. I love caffeine, but I'm not going to take expensive pills when I can just drink coffee and get the same effect.

While caffeine can have a low-grade fat-burning effect, where it really shines is in exercise performance. If you want to experiment, consume your caffeinated beverage of choice about thirty minutes before you hit the gym. Caffeine also has an appetite-blunting effect on some people, which is the main reason many people who use the Leangains method of IF start their day with a cuppa joe. Coffee to get you going and suppress your appetite, then lunch and dinner as usual.

> Just slow down on the caffeine intake later in the day. One of the most amazing things you can do to get your body to agree with your efforts to lose fat is to get consistent sleep.

Now let's talk about some other supplements you may want to consider if you want to optimize. Please note that we're at the tippy top of that diet pyramid of importance here, and that there are no supplements that will make any real difference if you're not doing right by the lower levels of the pyramid.

First up is creatine monohydrate. Creatine is the most studied supplement in the world when it comes to increasing gym performance. What it does is supply your cells with the raw materials necessary for rapid energy production in the mitochondria (the "power plant of the cell," as you probably learned in 9th-grade biology).

What this means in real life in the gym is that you can often squeeze out an extra rep or three when doing your final sets of an exercise. Those extra reps can add up over the months, which can eventually lead to more muscle gain.

Now, I know that this book is about fat loss, but creatine can help you with muscle retention while you are practicing your necessary calorie deficit. You just need to add one other ingredient: iron. As in, the kind of iron you pump.

Plain old creatine monohydrate is the best, so don't spend money on some of the other more expensive forms out there. And you also don't need to "load" creatine like the label will probably tell you to do (because they want you to take a whole lot up front so you'll run out of it faster). It doesn't need to be consumed just before working out or anything like that. Just take five grams a day at whatever time of day you prefer.

One last note on creatine: If you're not lifting weights there's not much call to add creatine to your arsenal. It should also be noted that some people are considered "non-responders" to creatine. In short, they can take it and not notice an effect. There's only one way to find out if that's you. Since creatine is not a steroid, is not in any way habit-forming, and not hard on your kidneys, to mention three of the top concerns on the internet about it, there's no reason not to give it a try.

Next up are protein supplements. I'll be the first to tell you that getting your protein from your meals is the best way to go, but I also admit that it's sometimes hard to hit my protein target for the day without supplementing.

There are many types of protein powders out there. Whey protein has been studied long and hard, and has many advantages when trying to increase your muscle mass. Whey's cousin, casein, is more slowly digested and will last long after whey is done. In reality, it doesn't matter that much. I just like the taste of what I take, which happens to be a whey/casein combo.

Again, supplementing your protein is not absolutely necessary but may be helpful either as a meal replacement or just another way to increase your total protein intake for the day. Whey and casein will give you the best bang for your buck, but some of the other types out there can be helpful too. Just keep your eye on the label, track everything, and test your results.

Next on the hit parade are vitamins and minerals, including my favorite supplement for the general population: vitamin D. Taking vitamin D will not make your belly fat fall off, but having low vitamin D is associated with all kinds of things you don't want, such as increased risk of cancer and cardiac disease. Vitamin D is also cheap. Optimizing your vitamin D levels can help fine-tune your immune system, improve your cognitive health, keep your bones strong and healthy, and if you're a dude, help keep your testosterone levels where they belong. For best results, get your blood tested to see where your D level is, and then talk to your doctor about supplementation. I have been taking 5,000 IU every day for years. I recently had some blood work done, and it showed my D levels were in the sweet spot.

Just behind vitamin D is another popular supplement that deserves your consideration. Fish oil, or more specifically docosahexaenoic acid (DHA) and eicosapentaenoic acid (EPA), are anti-inflammatory, heart-protective, and can help lower your body's triglycerides. I recommend getting a 250-500 mg (milligrams) combination of EPA and DHA every day. I love fish but I don't eat it that often, so I supplement. If you happen to eat a lot of cold-water fish, however, I wouldn't bother.

I would assume some of you have already heard of vitamin D and fish oil, but my next recommendation is sometimes new to people: magnesium.

Magnesium is a part of the energy production system of your body. You need it for the contraction and relaxation of muscle tissue. Magnesium is also helpful in maintaining insulin sensitivity which helps stave off diabetes. Low magnesium levels can cause elevated blood pressure and are also associated with symptoms of depression and ADHD. Magnesium has a paradoxical effect: although it helps with your energy production system, it also enables you to relax. Many people report sleeping better when they start using a magnesium supplement. In addition, it's one of the few supplements that people can feel working within a day or so of taking it.

Magnesium is an essential mineral that you get from your diet, but most people don't get optimal levels from diet alone. If you eat a lot of leafy greens and nuts you're probably all right on magnesium, but I use a supplement myself because I'm looking for "optimal," not just "good enough." There are many forms of magnesium supplementation, but I recommend either citrate or glycinate to the tune of 200-400 mg a day. The only real downside to magnesium supplementing is gastrointestinal upset if you take too much, so start on the low side and work your way up to 400.

There are a couple of other supplements I want to mention, but they are condition-specific.

Condition one: low testosterone in men. If this is you, you may want to consider taking a zinc supplement. Before you do that, talk to your doctor. If you eat red meat you're probably good on zinc, and low testosterone tends to be a many-sided problem. The sweet spot for supplementation is between 5 and 45 mg a day.

Condition two: arterial stiffness from calcification. If you have any kind of arterial calcification you may want to supplement with 200 mcgs (micrograms) of vitamin K-2 every day. Vitamin K helps direct the calcium ions to your bones and out of your arteries and soft tissues, helping to avoid calcification. Caution—don't take vitamin K if you're on a blood thinner, like Warfarin.

> There's a heart test called the Coronary Calcium Scan where you get a picture of your heart taken by CT, which can show any calcification. It's a fantastic test for predicting risk of a coronary event, and it only takes a few minutes to get it done. If you're over 40, it's a good idea to know your score.

We've now scaled the pyramid, ending with the least important piece of the puzzle, supplements. Now, let's talk about the practical implications when it comes to applying all this information to real life.

ELEVEN
Strategies for the Daily Grind

You now know all you need to start your journey toward weight loss the right way, based on your food preferences and with as much dietary freedom as you can have, while still making progress. One of the hard parts about fat loss is that we all want it yesterday. That's the reason people jump on a treadmill and start trying to run it off. It feels like something positive is happening at the time. They get sweaty and hot, and it feels like they just might be melting some fat right off. But the fact is that fat loss is a waiting game that is won in the kitchen much more than in the gym.

That being said, it's important to talk through some strategies based on your particular personality. After all, we're all different. For example, some people have no problem with rigorously tracking their calorie intake but others, when faced with the idea of tracking and measuring and such, would rather give up before they even get started. But I'm afraid that no matter your personality type, you're going to have to spend some amount of time quantifying your dietary intake. My suggestion is that you weigh and measure the food you eat for at least one month minimum. It's the only accurate way to become "calorically aware."

But here's the good news: the more you track, the easier it gets to keep tracking. Any of the popular tracking apps out there will remember your most commonly eaten foods. And let's face it, most of us eat the same ten things over and over. Once you've tracked your food intake for a week, you'll start inputting items based on your history a lot more often than having to look up new food items all the time.

This initial phase of tracking helps you start getting some momentum going. And one of the most important things I can tell you about finding success with fat loss is that it's momentum, not motivation, that wins the long race.

If you happen to have the "I hate to track" mindset, you may find that you love the results you see a lot more than you hate to track. You will also find that as you gain experience with paying more attention to the caloric details you will slowly become better at eating intuitively; that is, naturally choosing low calorie items without having to look them up.

The people who want to be more calorie-intuitive often find that one of the IF strategies works for them. But a word of caution— it's still easy to overconsume calories even on a restricted eating schedule, especially if you eat out often.

Eating out regularly can be a considerable obstacle for fat loss. The calorie density of restaurant food is almost always higher than what's reported. If you have a sales job or some other type of work that forces you to eat out, it can be helpful to read the menu ahead of time and make a plan. Many of the tracking apps can give you a ballpark estimate of different menu items. Just try and minimize the damage and take it easy at dinner when you get home later. You will still make progress.

And progress, not perfection, is the name of the game. No matter your personality type, you will find that being flexible and allowing yourself to indulge in small portions of less than ideal foods (for me it's ice cream or some kind of dessert) will enable you to keep moving forward without succumbing to the binge behavior that is so common when following super-restrictive diets.

What happens is that you'll establish a rhythm over the months where you are making steady improvements. As all of this becomes a habit, it will get easier to keep making progress until you start getting really lean. And it won't feel like torture because you've been eating foods on your list of preferred foods.

Speaking of lists of preferred foods, I want to take a moment to talk about the satiety index, or how much appetite satisfaction a particular food can give you, and how it can help you eat less without even thinking about it. This is especially helpful for the "I hate to track" crowd.

Back in 1995 researchers did a test of 38 different foods from six different categories (fruits, bakery products, snack foods, carbohydrate-rich foods, protein-rich foods, and breakfast cereals) to determine how filling each type of food was. Participants ate foods from the list and were later allowed to eat from a buffet of broader choices. The less they ate at the buffet indicated how filling the pre-buffet food was.

The number one, undisputed and unexpected champion of appetite satisfaction, was the boiled white potato. On the graph, which is readily available on the internet, it stands so much higher than everything else that it looks like it was shot out of a cannon. Take that, low-carb zealots.

> Just Google "satiety index" to see the graph with all the foods that were tested and how they ranked.

Other foods high on the satiety index were fish and other protein-rich foods, fibrous vegetables, eggs, oatmeal, and foods that are high-volume but lower-calorie like lettuce. Apples and oranges were the two most filling fruits. The lowest score on the list were croissants, with cakes, doughnuts, and candy bars falling in right behind them. No surprise, really, but it does support the idea that the more minimally processed foods you eat the easier it will be to stay full and not be tempted to overeat later.

Managing your appetite is the most obvious shortcut to losing body fat and eating more of the foods that are both calorie-poor and nutritionally rich is an obvious strategy. But eating less of the trigger foods, those items that we have a hard time stopping once we start, is another major obstacle when it comes to getting lean and mean.

To that end, we need to talk about your food environment—your pantry and fridge. One of the easiest ways to avoid your personal trigger foods is to make it inconvenient to get to them in the first place. Sometimes putting your trigger foods out of reach is all it takes to eat less of them, so if you have to get in the car and drive somewhere at 8:30 at night to eat some crackers, well, you'll probably skip the temptation.

> Of course, sometimes I'll get in the car and drive through somewhere for ice cream. But since that's a major hassle, it's also a self-limiting behavior.

Another handy strategy I use all the time is the 20-minute rule. It goes like this: If I want to snack, especially if I've recently eaten, like right after dinner, I make myself wait twenty full minutes before indulging to make sure I'm truly hungry and not just bored or looking to food for comfort. If I make it the full twenty minutes and still want the snack, I allow myself to have it. You would be amazed how often that 20-minute buffer keeps me out of the pantry.

Speaking of snacking, you may want to consider not doing it at all. For many people the simple act of only eating at mealtimes can make a huge difference. It is way too easy to eat more than you realize or want to admit if you nibble from a bowl of treats at the office. When I was finishing school, I once did an internship where they had a jar full of animal crackers in the break room. Every day I would stop by and grab a small handful. I was wearing scrubs with drawstring pants for this internship, which was a dangerous thing because I couldn't tell that my waistline was expanding by the week. A few weeks before my graduation I tried on the pants that I planned to wear for the event and was shocked to see how tight they had gotten, all from a single daily handful of animal crackers.

The truth is that a nibble here and a nibble there means suddenly you've eaten 4-500 extra calories in a day that you haven't accounted for, and those calories do indeed count. So to that end, consider making a "no snack" rule for yourself and see how it goes.

Your body doesn't care what time of the day you eat your food. There is no magic moment where everything you eat gets stored as fat. That being said, if you're unwilling to track your daily intake for the long term, you may consider having an evening cutoff time where you don't allow yourself to eat any more food. Just because I like to go to bed with a full belly doesn't mean you have to. Some people do well by sleeping through their hunger instead of experiencing it during the day.

Cutoff times can be a strategy that will help shape your behavior and habits to align with your goal of weight loss. There is no reason to live in fear of the clock striking 8 pm and feeling like anything you eat after that will turn you into a pumpkin. You can break the rule if the situation calls for it by paying attention to how much you eat earlier in the day, to give yourself the wiggle room to eat later that night if you want to.

About "cheating" on your diet: The awesome thing about this flexible dieting approach is that you get to make your own rules based on your strengths and weaknesses around food. It the "not a diet" diet. You're eating foods you like, but within reasonable limits based on your goals.

When you coast into your desired body fat level, it's much easier to camp out there because there's no diet to end. But if you've been "going keto" or some other fad diet for six months and can't wait for the day you can eat french fries again, you've been setting yourself up for gorging and weight regain. However, if you've been allowing yourself the occasional indulgence while keeping track of it and making steady progress, there's no reason to "cheat." There's nothing to cheat from because you made your own rules when it comes to dietary choices, and you won't feel deprived of your favorites.

After tracking your daily intake for a month, you may want to start experimenting with the concept known as "intuitive eating." I don't think most people will be as successful with this approach as they would be with rigorous tracking, but I also know that most people are going to have times in their lives that make it hard to do much more than get by, because life will happen. And it can be hard. If you find life happening to you but you still want to manage your body fat levels and try to improve, I offer the following strategies:

One: If you're in the middle of one of the storms of life, forget the macros. Just try and manage your total calories. If you're in a smaller storm and you want to do a little more than only tracking calories, aim to hit your protein goal for the day while maintaining your calorie deficit. If you're not in any storm but just hate tracking and want to wean yourself off it, know that most people who try to not count calories but just eat more intuitively will fail at that a few times before they get the hang of it.

And since you're going to try it anyway, I offer the following suggestions for intuitive eating from my friend, fitness super-hero Bryan Krahn:

Learning the calorie counts of your favorite foods and tracking them is a highly effective fat-loss tool.

However, for sustainable, life-long success you need to learn to differentiate between what's true hunger and what's merely cravings, boredom, habit, etc.

Catch is, you can't master the latter unless you temporarily step away from the former.

But most people are unsuccessful at making the transition the first few times they try. Especially if their lives lack structure or they're under a lot of stress.

To make it easier, here are some tips:

◆ See "intuitive eating" as more of a challenge, something you try for a few months when you're "settled" and in the right frame of mind.

◆ Do not try it when you're swamped or stressed.

◆ Don't jump in too deep. Rather than just switching to "winging" your diet, start by "eyeballing" one meal a day and go from there.

◆ Evaluate! You should still keep some kind of account of what you eat every day (a running log on Notes for example) and evaluate how well you did (and your body composition) every few weeks.

◆ Think. The whole point of the transition is to learn to "hear" what your body is trying to tell you. Exercises like asking yourself "am I really hungry or just bored?" in response to cravings may sound childish but is very enlightening.

◆ Relax. If you're a hardcore tracker, you WILL have a few fumbles making the transition. You might even crash and burn more than once. And that's okay. Because you can always go back to tracking macros—that skill isn't going anywhere—and recapture any progress you might have lost.

The point is never to stop growing and learning to truly listen to your body is one of the most rewarding lessons of all.

Thanks, Bryan. Good stuff.

↳ Check out Bryankrahn.com to follow him, which you should do.

Like he said, you have to experiment with this stuff. Don't take a short-term increase in body fat as a defeat—see it as a data point that can further inform your game plan.

Another piece of the snack-time puzzle that can make a big difference for your calorie deficit is swapping your familiar high-calorie pantry fare for something that will still scratch the snack itch without using up very much of your daily calorie budget. Sometimes you just gotta scratch that snack itch. And it's the itch for snacking itself more than any specific snack food that will get the job done. So, have some very low-calorie snacks on hand to munch on to keep yourself from eating an entire box of high-calorie crackers. Mmmm, crackers. Once the snack itch gets scratched, you can go back to your binge watching or reading your book, or working, or doing whatever, without that voice in the back of your mind telling you to haunt the kitchen.

For example—I keep some powdered chocolate-flavored peanut butter on hand that has almost all the fat removed (there are several brands out there). Because of the lack of fat, this stuff is very low calorie. You add a little water to get the consistency you want, and, boom—instant tasty treat. I mix that stuff up and throw a low-carb tortilla in the oven (nothing against carbs, but low-carb tortillas crisp up better than the regular ones). Add the sweet mix to the salty/crispy tortilla and I've got a delicious late-night snack that's around 110 calories and does virtually no damage to my calorie deficit.

Even better—if you like the taste of sushi, or more specifically, the nori seaweed used in making standard sushi rolls, there are packs of nori crisps that come in different flavors (I'm a wasabi man myself) that scratch that salty/crunchy itch nicely. And an entire pack of them is only 15-ish calories.

Of course, my tastes aren't necessarily yours, but the point is that finding substitutes for your more calorie-dense go-to snacks can make it a lot less painful to maintain your calorie deficit.

Another strategy you might consider is substituting sparkling water for soft drinks. Soft drinks are a hidden source of calories that many people don't even consider when it comes to tracking their daily food intake. There is no shortage of flavored waters on the market, and the longer I drink them, the more overpowering a regular soda seems when I have a sip. Kicking a soda habit can be a significant win for you.

One last tip: Most people are going to be way off on their estimates about two things—how much weight they need to lose to get the look they want, and how long it will take them to get there. So be patient, and don't be afraid to reevaluate your thinking as you go along. The days are long in this game, but the months go by quickly, and in no time, you'll be a whole new you.

TWELVE
After the Diet: Where the Real Work Begins

Most people can lose weight when they try, and as hard as losing weight can be, it's far from the hardest part. The ultimate challenge is keeping the weight off once you get to your weight-loss destination.

One of the advantages of the flexible dieting approach is that there is no rigid diet to go off of when you get to your target body. "Being done" with a diet is the single biggest reason people regain the weight they lost, and more. Going back to the same old eating habits that put on the weight in the first place is an excellent way to gain everything back, lose the progress, and render the dietary sacrifices you've made useless.

The human body is designed to store fat in times of famine as a safety mechanism. After an extended time living in a caloric deficit, your body will be more primed than ever to gain fat in preparation for the next perceived "famine" of another calorie deficit.

Because of this fat storage reflex, you must proceed with caution once you hit your target weight, which will hopefully not be too painful since you've already been eating according to your preferences to get there in the first place. But once you get there, you must resist the idea that you can have a gorge-fest to celebrate.

The fact is, by the end of an extended calorie deficit, your testosterone is low (if you're a guy), and your cortisol (a stress hormone) levels are elevated. Ghrelin, a hormone that stimulates appetite, will be elevated, and leptin, a hormone that helps you feel full and stop eating, will be low.

But hey, at least you look fantastic at the pool, right?

Once you get to your desired weight, the trick is to slowly increase calories from either carbs, fats, or a combination of the two to start recalibrating your hormones and send the signal that you're no longer in a "famine" state, but without so many added calories that you start packing on too much fat again.

And by slowly, I mean, like, really slowly.

This so-called reverse dieting is one of the areas where the die-hard trackers will shine. The amount of food you're going to be adding each week will be very small, so the more accurately you can track small amounts the better off you'll be when it comes to finding your new maintenance calorie level. My suggestion is to add no more than 200 calories a day per week. I know. That's nothing. It's a light snack, at best. And you should make it just a light snack, so you give yourself the feeling of adding something extra to your daily intake. Make it feel special.

When you're reverse dieting up to your maintenance level it's a good idea to weigh yourself daily and calculate a weekly average. You can expect your scale to fluctuate daily, especially if you're adding carbs back to a low-carb diet. Another thing you should be doing at least once a week during the reverse dieting phase is measuring your waistline.

If you've been restricting calories for a while, and have been hitting the gym, you'll start to notice the weights getting a little lighter and your overall sense of well-being blossoming. Take that as evidence that your cortisol levels are returning to normal, and if you're a guy, your testosterone levels are increasing, too.

Normalizing your body's cortisol level by reverse dieting will make it easier to maintain the look you've worked so hard to achieve. When you feel good and have made progress by ditching the fad diets and sticking to the flexible dieting method, your body will respond in kind by slowly allowing you to eat more without it all going into fat storage.

Eventually, you'll get to a point where you've slowly ramped up your calories to find your "true maintenance" level, which will be higher than the caloric intake you used to get to your current desired weight. The refeed strategy, while not for everyone, can be a useful tool to hit the reset switch on your hormones and your sanity, while giving you an extra boost in the gym for a few workouts.

And finally, I know I've been talking about how important your food choices are for losing the weight. And they are. But the "energy out" part of the equation seems to be the important part for keeping the weight off once you get there. A study from 2019 entitled "Physical Activity Energy Expenditure and Total Daily Energy Expenditure in Successful Weight Loss Maintainers"[1] found that people who have the most success keeping the weight off long term have the highest energy expenditure—they willingly burned more calories through exercise. So, find something you like, or at least that you don't hate, and start doing it while you're getting better at the tracking and calorie restriction part of this game.

> Seriously, the key here is finding something that you can slowly fall in love with when it comes to exercise. I personally like lifting weights because it's easy to track progress, it gives me the look I want, and I get to do it in the air-conditioned gym. Hey, it's hot in Houston, Texas. Some people love to run or cycle or swim. Just find your thing and start falling in love with it.

Almost every person I've ever spoken to (and that's a lot of people) who has lost a lot of weight and kept it off has one thing in common. They all consider themselves "fit people," and a part of their identity is their "fitness life." Fitness became a part of their working definition of themselves. Think of the most fit person you know and think about that for a moment and you'll see that it's true.

So, the best formula for permanent weight loss is calorie restriction while finding an exercise routine you like at the same time. Get to your goal weight and reverse diet until you find your maintenance. Then shift your focus to the "energy out" part of the equation by falling more in love with your exercise selection.

Do all of these things with some planning and diligence, and you can eat pie and such at Christmastime and still fit into your pants with no problem.

---

1   https://www.ncbi.nlm.nih.gov/pubmed/30801984

THIRTEEN
Fad Diets, Detoxes, and Cleanses

Let's take a minute to look at some of the more popular trends in the weight-loss industry. Knowing what we know now, we can peek behind the curtain and get a feel for why they work and what their limitations are compared to the flexible dieting approach I've been advocating in this book. The key to them all, as you will see, is that they put you in a calorie deficit, often without you even knowing it. Once people have some success (and the initial success with many of these diets is only water weight), they become hardcore converts to the philosophy.

But you're not going to be as easily tricked, because now you know the rules: calorie deficit is king, protein is satiating and also necessary when it comes to muscle mass retention, and everything else is just details.

Let's start with the biggest of today's buzzwords: keto.

"Keto" stands for the ketogenic diet, which is an extremely low-carb diet that supposedly melts fat off your body because, as its adherents will tell you over and over again, "when you don't eat carbs your body will start burning fat as fuel." True believers dip test strips in their urine to make sure they are in true ketosis, the state your body enters when there is inadequate glucose available for fuel. Keep in mind that glucose is the preferred fuel source for your brain and nervous system as well as your muscles when it comes to healthy functioning.

So, do keto (and other low-carb diets) work? Sure. Does it work because you're shutting down insulin production and somehow becoming more efficient by using ketones for fuel? Nope.

Let's mentally walk through the process when someone "goes keto." Step one: Read a bunch of stuff on the internet about how magical it is, and that you get to eat as much steak and eggs as you want. It's also supposed to work really fast—many people report dropping close to ten pounds in their first couple of weeks. Our hero thinks he only needs to lose about ten pounds to begin with, so why not make it a fun adventure that gets him to his goal faster?

Off to the store to buy loads of steak and eggs. And sausage. And bacon. Maybe some deli meat and cheese. Wow, that was a quick trip to the grocery store because you're not allowed to eat much more than that (rule one: if you burn more calories than you consume, you'll lose weight). Do you see where we're going with this yet?

Our keto experimenter starts day one by adding a bunch of butter to his coffee 'cause the internet told him that would be a good idea. And, whoa, he has so much more energy than usual—the internet told him he would, and it's true! For lunch, our hero eats a bag of tuna and half an avocado. What else is there that he can eat? He needs to get on a keto forum and get some more ideas. Dinner is steak and eggs. It's awesome. He'd been thinking about that all day.

Wash, rinse, repeat. A week goes by, and our man steps on the scale. Five pounds down already. This is easy! So easy, in fact, that our man starts telling everyone he knows about keto. He is now a Keto Warrior (KW).

Week two yields similar results. The weigh-in after a mere 14 days shows a ten-pound drop in weight, right on the money. Our KW is outwardly ecstatic. But only outwardly. Here's what's going on inwardly: "Ten pounds went fast, but I can barely tell a difference in my love handles or belly fat."

"Last week I felt stronger than this week—and last week I could lift more weight or do more reps on just about every lift in the gym."

"I'm sick of eating the same five things over and over again. And is consuming all this fat really good for me? And will I ever get to eat real pizza again?"

"Ketosis-breath is not good for interpersonal relations."

And, a personal favorite: "It seems as though I could use some fiber in my diet these days."

Meanwhile, on a deep level, a low-grade fear of eating carbs is starting to develop. The same carbs, by the way, that would be great for fueling the body to have better workouts and better clarity of mind.

Let's look at what really goes on in your standard keto diet so we can get back to the fundamentals of how fat loss really works instead of looking for a magic bullet solution like the keto diet.

First on the hit parade when starting keto: loss of water weight. Like, a lot of water weight. Inside your body carbs convert to glucose, which is stored as glycogen in your liver and your muscle tissue, where it gets used for fuel. Each gram of glycogen binds to 3-4 grams of water. Your average person stores around one pound of glycogen. Your average overweight person? They may have more than a pound. It can be double the average for some people. Double the glycogen storage means double the water storage, too.

Let's say you have two pounds of glycogen stored pre-keto. That two pounds is holding onto eight total pounds of water. Then you go keto and use up all that stored glycogen. When the glycogen stores go, the water goes with it, and presto, ten pounds lost without any change in fat storage.

But it sure looks cool on the scale. And that initial drop can be motivating to keep going (and to become a keto advocate online). But once the water storage dries up and the scale's momentum slows down, there can be trouble in paradise. And trouble usually means one of two things:

1. A binge, or
2. Doubling down on keto.

Funny thing about the binge version—the ten pounds returns overnight, but the binger doesn't wake up looking any different. Often the binge is on delicious, carby things that have been off limits, and the body's glycogen stores are refilled. The body gets its favorite fuel source again, and if the binger feels enough guilt to hit the gym the next day they will often experience an uptick in performance. Heavy weights get lighter. The last few reps come easier. The race car has fuel (glucose) again.

But for the double-down keto warrior the answer might well be to eat less protein and more fat. Why? Because protein can be turned into glucose in times of desperate need. So they think, I've been eating a lot of protein in lieu of carbs, but my body is making carbs from the protein. So, I'll eat more fat instead.

The keto warrior is now very likely to have the following train of events occur: They will eat way too much saturated fat, which can have an adverse effect on cholesterol and triglyceride levels. In fact, a 2019 study[2] compared keto to non-keto for changes in blood lipids (cholesterol) and inflammation, and after four weeks on keto the participants' markers for both had increased significantly from their baseline measurements.

I stumbled across this study about a week before meeting with my publisher, but I had written the first sentence of that paragraph long before the meeting. Yay, science!

In extreme cases, rare but still worth mentioning, the body can enter a state of keto-acidosis where the blood chemistry gets too acidic. In this situation, minerals are pulled from the bones as a buffer to keep the blood pH in check. Last time I checked, brittle bones aren't cool.

And this is all in the name of becoming "fat-burning adapted," which is largely a myth. The body needs fuel, and in the absence of glucose, it'll work with whatever it has to work with to keep metabolic function moving along. But as I have mentioned before, there's a big difference between "getting by" and "optimal." And when you're trying to lift heavy weights or cycle or run fast, you want optimal.

2   https://www.ncbi.nlm.nih.gov/pubmed/31067015

Still, people do lose weight on a ketogenic diet. Here's why: They are eating fewer calories than they are using. Often much less, because people get sick of eating the same few things over and over. They end up eating less and less, until they finally give up on the whole thing and go back to what they really want to do, which is to eat carbs again.

Often, the keto warrior who starts slipping a little on protocol has the most success. The carbs that have crept back into their diet will fuel better training sessions and more serotonin release at night, which makes for better sleep. Better sleep makes for better body composition even without doing anything else to lose weight. So will better training sessions.

You know what you call the ketogenic diet with added carbs? Sustainable (and no longer keto). Because in a calorie deficit with high protein intake something has to go: carbs, fats, or a combination. I suggest finding what works best for you, given your food preferences and training intensity. One more suggestion: Most people find they can eat less fat and be okay with it since fat is more calorically dense than carbs. However, dietary fat doesn't do much for hard workouts in the gym.

Now let's turn the lens away from low-carbs and keto and onto another current fad diet that again, often works for people, but again may not be working for the reasons that people claim. And it's definitely more work than necessary in order to see the needle drop in your favor.

That diet is The Whole 30.

Now the rage shall flow for many reading this but hear me out. I've done ten days of TW30 myself. Ten miserable, long days that made me start hating sweet potatoes and avocados, which I've always loved. Let's review the basics. TW30 is billed as a way to reset your diet with a focus on whole foods. They claim that adherents will heal their guts, reduce systemic inflammation, and restore their healthy metabolism. What's not to love?

What distinguishes TW30 is what you can't eat, contained in a short list which consists of anything that brings joy and happiness:

- No sugar.

- No alcohol.
- No grains (which means nothing crunchy).
- No legumes, or dairy, or baked goods or candy, pizza, tacos, or fun.

But at least there's an end to it: thirty days.

And that, my friend, is one of its major problems. Thirty days? You could stand on your head for thirty days if you had to, but that doesn't mean you will have learned anything life-changing. Like I've said previously in this book—real change is about changing your everyday habits, not just enduring a month of eating from a small list of foods that you may or may not like.

Before I bash TW30 much further, let me talk about what I do like about it.

The emphasis on whole foods is laudable. Who would be against people eating more unprocessed, minimally refined foods? And there's a lot of encouragement for people to get back into the kitchen and fall in love with cooking again. One of the most important steps you can take to improve your health and waist measurement is to start cooking more of your own food, and that's part of TW30.

TW30 tends to make people default to eating a higher amount of protein to fill up, which will make eating fewer calories easier. The extra protein will also aid in muscle retention (and possibly building some new muscle) if the dieter is hitting the gym, which they should be doing. In other words, a diet which is higher in protein intake is going to be generally more successful than one that isn't. Sound familiar?

However—TW30 is to the "paleo diet" as keto is to "Atkins." There is truly nothing new under the sun. And, like the paleo diet and its other derivatives, the biggest problem has to do with the categorization of major food groups into "good" and "bad" categories.

There are foods that can cause problems in some people, and for those people avoiding foods on TW30s no-no list makes sense. But putting things like dairy and grains into the bad camp for thirty days can make people with no sensitivity to those foods paranoid about eating them again.

Often, the perceived bogeyman with these foods is inflammation. Now, I'm not going to tell you that your dietary choices won't affect the level of inflammatory markers in your body. But I'm also not going to tell you that eating beans or drinking alcohol or chowing down any of the other off-limits foods from TW30 is going to light up your inflammatory markers like the Scarecrow in a forest fire. The fact is that you can lower your levels of inflammation simply by reducing your body fat levels.

Don't forget Mark Haub, who lost 27 pounds eating Twinkies and other assorted gas station fare throughout a semester when he wanted to prove to his students that calories are king when it comes to weight loss. By the end of his experiment, he'd dropped 4% of his body fat. He also saw an increase of his HDL cholesterol by about 20%, a decrease of his LDL cholesterol by 20%, and a decrease in his triglycerides by 39%. All of these markers are indicators of lowering inflammation. To be fair, he did include a protein shake every day of this diet. But the vast majority of his caloric intake came from food that is as about as anti-TW30 as you can get.

Now, neither Haub nor I am going to tell you that eating crap from the gas station is a great long-term solution to your dieting woes. But I am going to tell you, again, that eating to your preferences is going to give you the best likelihood of long-term success.

By the way, I think TW30 might be a good way to help figure out if you have any actual food sensitivities, because doing TW30 is essentially doing an elimination diet. Many people claim that their skin clears up and that they have less gas and bloating after making it through the thirty days. I couldn't tell you whether this is true, since I was ready to lose my mind after ten days. But I think that there's enough power of suggestion going around on TW30 message boards to influence people's thinking about it.

So. TW30. Inasmuch as it directs people toward nutritionally dense whole foods, I'm for it. Inasmuch as it makes people scared to eat foods that they ordinarily have no issues with, I'm not for it. TW30 doesn't teach you how to learn to love the process of making the change. It teaches you how to endure short-term suffering for a short-lived reward. The short-term nature of TW30 steers people into an "it's only thirty days" mentality instead of teaching them how to build lifetime habits that involve the preferences they (you!) can truly own to achieve long-lasting success.

Instead of trying thirty days of complete, radical change I'd suggest thirty days of tracking your daily intake instead, so you can become more calorically aware about the foods you already eat. Maybe you could figure out a few substitutes for some of the higher calorie foods you eat more regularly, and then buckle in for a lifetime of changed habits that will put you on a path you enjoy. The real change comes from learning to enjoy the journey.

You know what else doesn't prepare you for long-term, sustainable success? "Detoxes" and "cleanses." I put those words in quotes because they don't really mean what they imply.

Many of the fad diets that come and go claim to detoxify your body and reset it to be a better fat burner, cure your gut, reduce inflammation, and more. And it's all a waste of time. Almost without exception, adherents of detoxes can never tell you what kind of toxins they are getting rid of. But boy, do they feel better for having done one. Cleansers never know what they've cleaned out but it doesn't stop them from telling everyone they know about how awesome cleanses are.

Take, for instance, the Master Cleanse. This one makes the rounds every few years, it seems. The plan is that you eat nothing, and drink nothing but lemon juice with a little maple syrup and cayenne pepper for ten days. Since there's no fiber being consumed during the cleanse, there's a handy "cleansing tea" you can drink to assist you in having a bowel movement. And by "bowel movement," I mean "white knuckle, full body clenching, emptying of the cellar." Please understand that kind of movement isn't eliminating toxins, but it probably is the closest you'll come to having a stroke that day.

When people pull off any of the popular cleanses and detoxes, they are really just eliminating most, if not all, of their usual caloric intake for the days that they do it. Glycogen stores in the body get depleted. Water weight is lost. The scale can go down quickly, but temporarily. And again, no new lifelong habits are formed. It's basically suffering for the sake of suffering, where no real fat loss occurs.

Every other decade or so a variation of the "cabbage soup diet" sweeps across the land. If you haven't heard of it yet, just wait. Adherents claim they can lose weight and detoxify their bodies by eating nothing but cabbage soup for however long they can stand to.

The fact is, the combination of marketing and social media hype that happens with these fads makes them seem irresistible to people who "just need to lose ten pounds." Not to mention that as long as you have a normally functioning set of kidneys and your liver is still in there somewhere, you have all the mechanisms in place to detoxify your body just fine.

I haven't been immune to the pull of "just ten pounds" myself over the years. Long before I took the deep dive into the research that led me to write this book, I succumbed to the temptation to drop ten pounds quickly. Like, more than once.

I once followed the Atkins Diet for around a month. I lost ten pounds very quickly and then gained them right back. And I have to admit—watching the weight on the scale drop that fast was supremely motivating. While it lasted. I also must admit that I wanted to eat a potato so badly during that time that I dreamed about it. In the end, I did lose some fat on a very low-carb diet because I was getting so sick of eating the same few things over and over that I eventually started eating less overall. But then the holidays came around, and pie entered the equation. I'm sure you can guess how that went.

Next on the list of fad diets I've personally explored is Sugar Busters. Sugar Busters became a thing in the mid-'90s. It doesn't take too much imagination to come up with the central tenet of that diet: SUGAR BAD.

On top of sugar being verboten, one must also avoid high glycemic index foods including high GI fruits like bananas and pineapple. Never mind that the GI has been shown not to matter at all when it comes to losing weight. But on the Sugar Busters diet I did start paying more attention to the quality of food I was eating. And I did lose weight, just like pretty much anyone who starts paying more attention to the foods they eat. Ultimately, I quit the Sugar Busters diet because it was too restrictive, and that was before I understood the research when it comes to the glycemic index. And sometimes, you just want to eat some ice cream.

And sometimes you just want to eat pizza. Pizza is the reason I decided to get off the horse when it comes to the Paleo Diet. Oh, I was full-on Paleo Guy for a while. It just made so much sense. Honestly, the way I eat from day to day now isn't too far removed from Paleo, with the exception that I still eat legumes and the occasional slice of bread.

But like TW30, Paleo puts way too many foods in the "bad" camp without considering the context of the average person who just needs to drop some weight. If someone thinks the only way they can be healthy and lose some fat is to give up grains, dairy, and vegetables from the nightshade family, well, they may just decide to stay fat and happy instead.

But if that person is told to eat a little more protein and a little less of everything else but could still eat the foods they like, then the prospect of stripping off some chub isn't as intimidating. Once the average person sees that more nutrient-dense foods like vegetables are also the lowest calorie choices, they will often start moving in that dietary direction naturally.

Add in some strength training to go along with the calorie deficit, and suddenly our hero has two markers of progress—gains in the gym and losses on the scale—all without resorting to diet extremes that the average person can never maintain for the long haul.

Be a hero. Don't get caught up in the hype that surrounds the fads and trends in the dieting world.

EPILOGUE
Bullet-Point Summary

H ere we are. You've made it to the end of this book, and you just got firehosed with a lot of information. Sometimes it's hard to think through it all and make an actual plan. So, here's your plan in handy-dandy bullet-point format:

- Calories count, so for as long as you can stand to do it you should count them to understand where you're truly at on how much you're eating and how much you should be eating.

- Beware—people suck at estimating and keeping track of how much they eat. Understand that up front, and try to get better at it. A food scale can be helpful when trying to understand portion sizes.

- There are many useful tracking apps for your phone. Explore the possibilities and use whatever one you prefer. Most of them will use the same formula as in this book for determining your calorie needs and will save you from doing some math.

- Protein is magical when it comes to keeping you full and preserving muscle mass when you're in a calorie deficit. You want to shoot for one gram of protein per pound of your desired body weight if you have more than 20 lbs. to lose, and one gram per pound of actual body weight if you have less than twenty pounds to drop. Instead of overeating all the time you will suddenly find that it is hard to eat enough in a day.

◆ After setting your daily protein intake level, the rest of your intake will come from carbs and fats. You'll have to lower one or both of them to create your calorie deficit. If you're sedentary, a lower-carb plan will be a better fit, since carbs are fuel for activity and you're not getting that much. If you plan on hitting the gym regularly (and I think you should, but that's another book) then consider dropping your fat intake and eating more carbs.

◆ Fad diets use black-and-white thinking and bastardized views of dietary science to sell you stuff. Don't buy into it. Most of the positive health changes people see from fad diets are simply due to the weight loss from consuming less food overall, not the actual diet itself.

◆ Carbs are not the enemy. Don't believe the hype. Neither is insulin. It's way more complicated than that, but at the same time it's as simple as eating less (but even that is complicated because we're all human and have different stressors in our lives that influence our eating behaviors).

◆ Low-carb diets mean you will drop many pounds in water weight. That can be great for getting some momentum going, but don't be fooled that it is fat loss. And don't be freaked out when you gain back that water weight when you start eating carbs again.

◆ If you're stressed just thinking about tracking your individual daily macros, then you can default to just lowering your total calories for the day. Your overall caloric intake is at the base of the diet pyramid for a reason: it's the part that makes the most significant difference. Macro tracking is more about optimizing, which can also be important, but not as much as total intake.

◆ Meal timing and frequency don't matter that much, so if you've been eating breakfast only because it's touted as "the most important meal of the day" you can consider skipping it and cutting those calories out of your daily intake.

◆ Carbs and protein are helpful to consume both before and after working out.

- You can absorb more than thirty grams of protein in one sitting.
- Supplements can be helpful for general health, but ones sold as fat burners are for the most part a complete waste of money.
- Don't buy into the idea that there are "clean" foods and "dirty" foods. You should eat the foods you prefer. Outside of any food allergies you might have, and trans fats, how much you eat is way more important than what you eat, once you consider your total calorie intake.
- Sticking to a diet that consists of the foods you actually like will make it way easier to stick to for the rest of your life.
- Take a diet break, and up your calories for a week or so every eight to ten weeks. Constant deprivation will crash your hormones and make you crazy. Once the break is over, get back on the horse and don't stress about the few pounds you gained on your break. They're mostly water weight, anyway.
- Once you get to your goal weight, you will see that your goals will have changed several times along the way. That's okay.
- Fat loss is not linear. You can be doing everything right and see no change in the scale for a week or more. Then you will have a week where the scale drops five to eight pounds. Expect it. Don't freak out. Give the process a chance.
- When you finally get to your target weight, don't lose your mind and binge more than one meal to celebrate. Now is the time to gradually increase your calories over several weeks by no more than about 200 calories per day per week. Even if you hate tracking, this is the time to do it anyway.
- Once you've gotten to your target weight and then slowly increased your daily calories, you'll hit your true maintenance number for caloric intake. It can take many weeks to get there, but it will be worth it to get there slow and easy. Rushing this stage after going on a diet is an excellent way to gain back a bunch of fat, because after your calorie-deficit stage your body is in "prepare for the next famine"

mode. The ongoing diet *after* your calorie-deficit diet is as important as the diet itself.

- Habits reign supreme. Habits can hurt you, but they can also help you. Short-term thinking is what gets people jumping from one fad diet to the next with no long-term results. Give yourself time, and adopt a set of habits and a long-term mindset toward your fat-loss goals.

- Finding snacking options that are lower-calorie substitutes for some of your favorites can be a good way to scratch the itch of the late-night snack without harming your weight loss goal.

- Strength training while dieting is the best way to preserve muscle mass and avoid the skinny-fat look. Muscle retention when you are in a daily calorie deficit means more fat is going to be lost by default. Something has to go, and if muscle retention is happening, there's nothing else to lose but your fat.

- Cardio is heart-healthy, as well as strength training. If you like cardio, do some cardio. I'm not discouraging it, but it is not nearly as impactful for muscle mass retention as strength training.

Finally—thanks for reading. I know there are roughly eleventy-billion diet books out there, and I'm grateful you spent some time with me here. Good luck, and good lifelong habits!

Notes

Readers can locate the articles cited in this book by going to the web site of the National Center for Biotechnology Information (NCBI) and typing the article title in the search box. When you search for the title it will give an abstract of the article. This is their URL: https://www.ncbi.nlm.nih.gov

For information on Martin Berkhan and his leangains method, visit his website: https://leangains.com

Made in the USA
Columbia, SC
13 August 2021